Rheumatoid Arthritis

and Related Diseases

Cover: The hand of a patient with rheumatoid arthritis (RA), showing metacarpophalangeal joint subluxation. This hand also illustrates multiple subcutaneous nodules, a characteristic in 20% to 30% of patients with progressive RA. *Reprinted from the* Clinical Slide Collection on the Rheumatic Diseases, *copyright 1991, 1995. Used by permission of the American College of Rheumatology.*

Rheumatoid Arthritis

and Related Diseases

Including:

- Rheumatoid Arthritis
- Chronic Fatigue Syndrome
- Fibromyalgia Syndrome
- Lupus Erythematosus
- Sjögren's Syndrome
- Systemic Sclerosis

Author:

ROBERT P. SUNDEL, MD

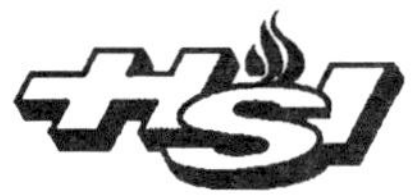

Health Studies Institute, Inc.

Rheumatoid Arthritis and Related Diseases

Printed in the United States of America
Incorporates material from *Connective Tissue Diseases* © 1993

Dr. Robert Picard Sundel, recognized as one of the foremost experts on Kawasaki disease, is equally respected for his work in immunology and rheumatology, especially among children. Dr. Sundel received his BA (*summa cum laude*) and his MD from Boston University. His postdoctoral training began with a residency in pediatrics at New York's Columbia-Presbyterian Medical Center Babies Hospital. Subsequently, he was a research associate in cellular immunology at the Hadassah Medical Center in Jerusalem and a fellow in allergy/immunology/rheumatology at Boston's Children's Hospital.

Dr. Sundel has remained at Children's Hospital since 1986. Among his responsibilities there have been service on ten committees including those on clinical research, quality improvement, clinical practice guidelines, medical student education, and internship selection. At present, he chairs the Program Review Committee on Intravenous Immunoglobulin, another of his research interests. He has been an attending physician in several programs and is Director of the Children's Hospital Rheumatology Program.

Additionally, since 1994, he has been assistant coordinator of Harvard Medical School's Pediatric Core Rotation at Children's Hospital. He is Medical Director and Service Chief of the Center for Ambulatory Treatment and Clinical Research at Children's Hospital, and serves on the Harvard Medical School faculty. He is a Fellow of both the American College of Rheumatology and the American Academy of Pediatrics.

In addition to holding state licenses from New York and Massachusetts, Dr. Sundel is a Diplomate of the American Board of Pediatrics, the American Board of Allergy & Immunology, and the Sub-board of Pediatric Rheumatology of the American Board of Pediatrics. He has received the Janeway Award for Excellence in Clinical Teaching from Children's Hospital, the ALPHA Therapeutic Award for contributions in the field of immunology, and the Adolescent Service Award for outstanding service to the Janeway Inpatient Medical Service. He serves on the Education Committee of the American Academy of Pediatrics, Section of Rheumatology, and on the Subcommittee in Juvenile Arthritis of the Arthritis Foundation of Massachusetts.

Dr. Sundel has published a number of journal articles on Kawasaki disease and on the treatment of juvenile rheumatoid arthritis, especially that involving intravenous immunoglobulin. He is an ad hoc reviewer for the *European Journal of Pediatrics, Arthritis & Rheumatism,* and *Pediatrics.* He continues to research Kawasaki disease, Lyme disease, pediatric arthritis, and therapeutic applications of intravenous gamma globulin, and to publish the results of his research in many journals and books.

Dr. Sundel attests that he has no actual or potential conflict of interest in relation to this book.

Special thanks to Faith S. Schaefer, BS, our senior staff writer, and Joan Schulman, MA, our senior staff editor, for their many contributions in developing this text.

Health Studies Institute
P.O. Box 6808
Deerfield Beach, FL 33442-6808

Contents

Algorithms

Color Plate

Black & White Illustrations

Tables of Information

Directions

How to Get the Most Out of This Course

Become completely familiar with the material in each chapter before going on to the next. First, preview by skimming the chapter, then read it. Study the tables, algorithms, illustrations, and appendices, and use the Definitions, Abbreviations, and Acronyms, and the Index in the back of the book to aid your understanding. Finally, quiz yourself, using the review questions between chapters to evaluate your mastery of the material. Go at your own pace.

The Post-Test

Please use a No. 2 pencil to fill out the answer form for the post-test. There are 50 questions; a passing grade requires 40 correct answers. Keep a copy of your answers for your own records. If you fail the post-test, you may retake it for a $5.00 service charge. Each question has only one correct answer; there are no trick questions and no deliberate fogginess. If you see a way to improve the questions, please note your suggestions on the certificate request form.

Certification

The purchase of a course entitles only one person, the named purchaser, to receive continuing education credit. If we don't have your name registered, we cannot send your certificate. We keep records for licensure and certification; please notify us if your name or address changes.

If you need a replacement certificate, we are glad to provide one. The replacement fee of $5 includes mailing and handling. Your state licensing board may request your certificate of completion, or a copy of it, so file it carefully.

Mailing Instructions

1. Make sure your name and the course title appear correctly on the post-test answer form.
2. Complete the certificate request form.
3. Mail both of these forms to: Health Studies Institute
   P.O. Box 6808
   Deerfield Beach, FL 33442-6808

We will mail your certificate promptly upon receipt of the answer form and certificate request. If you don't receive your certificate, please notify us: 1-800-700-3454. Thank you for continuing your professional education with us.

Health Studies Institute, Inc.

Objectives

At the end of this course, you will take a written test which will measure your ability to identify:

1. Signs and symptoms of four widespread rheumatic diseases <u>with</u> inflammation and autoimmunity:
   - Rheumatoid arthritis
   - Systemic lupus erythematosus
   - Sjögren's syndrome
   - Systemic sclerosis

2. Pathogenic features of autoimmunity and the above-mentioned rheumatic diseases

3. Signs and symptoms of two widespread forms of rheumatism <u>without</u> demonstrable inflammation or autoimmunity:
   - Chronic fatigue syndrome
   - Fibromyalgia syndrome

4. Diagnostic criteria for the six rheumatic diseases/syndromes discussed in this coursebook

5. The gender and ages of patients most often affected by these disorders.

6. Systemic manifestations associated with the six types of rheumatism.

7. Pharmacotherapies, their limitations, adverse side effects, and contraindications.

8. Nondrug therapies

9. Medical and blood tests used to identify and monitor affected patients.

Introduction

Most clinicians have at least one patient or know someone who suffers acute or chronic rheumatism. Perhaps you have observed:

- A 60-year-old patient who, because of temporomandibular joint pain, is unable to hold his mouth open for more than 30 seconds while receiving dental care *(see Chapter 1)*
- Your 30-year-old sister waking up exhausted after sleeping 8 hours, and hurting everywhere, just as she has for months *(see Chapter 2)*
- A 29-year-old co-worker who can't get a full night's sleep, and has unexplained generalized achiness, irritable bowel syndrome, and migraine headaches *(see Chapter 2)*
- A 30-year-old neighbor who no longer jogs because of his chest and toe pain, caused by pericarditis and microinfarcts *(see Chapter 3)*
- A 55-year-old friend whose dry tongue and painful caries prevent her from eating nutritious meals, and whose chapped lips are surrounded by perioral wrinkles *(see Chapter 4)*
- A 49-year-old aunt who, after suffering thickening and hardening of her skin for 3 years, dies of pulmonary interstitial fibrosis *(see Chapter 5)*.

This coursebook reviews six rheumatic diseases/syndromes which affect millions of people and can produce musculoskeletal pain and manifestations such as those described above.

Identification

Algorithm 1 shows important identifying clues to the six types of rheumatism discussed:

1. Rheumatoid arthritis, systemic lupus erythematosus, Sjögren's syndrome, and systemic sclerosis involve inflammation of and injury to joints, blood vessels, or connective tissue, and are generally regarded as autoimmune diseases. (*See Autoimmunity below.*)
2. Chronic fatigue syndrome and fibromyalgia syndrome produce pain and/or disabling fatigue, but without demonstrable inflammation or autoimmunity.

Algorithm 1. Identifying Six Rheumatic Disorders		
If a patient has:	**Consider:**	**Which most often affects:**
• Joint pain and morning stiffness • Deformed wrists • Joint swelling • Subcutaneous nodules • Symmetric, erosive synovitis	Rheumatoid arthritis (adult) *(See Chapter 1)*	• Females (the female-to male ratio is about 2.5:1) 30 to 60 years old • Persons >65 years old (either sex) most severely affected
• Fatigue (persistent and disabling) • Fever • Generalized achiness • Impaired cognition • Insomnia or hypersomnia	Chronic fatigue syndrome *(See Chapter 2)*	• Females (75% of patients are females) 18 to 45 years old
• Fatigue (persistent and disabling) • Sleep impairment • Tender point site pain • Widespread pain (often acute)	Fibromyalgia syndrome *(See Chapter 2)*	• Females (75% of patients are females) 20 to 50 years old
• Cutaneous signs (rash or lesions) • Fever and/or malaise • Nonerosive arthritis with arthralgia • Renal manifestations (common), or involvement of any organ system	Systemic lupus erythematosus *(See Chapter 3)*	• Non-White females (the female to male ratio is at least 5:1) 15 to 40 years old
• Keratoconjunctivitis sicca • Nonerosive arthritis with arthralgia • Xerostomia	Sjögren's syndrome *(See Chapter 4)*	• Females (90% of patients are females) 40 to 60 years old
• Flexion contractures of the hands • Itchy or uncomfortable skin tightening and thickening • Renal and pulmonary manifestations • Severe cold sensitivity	Systemic sclerosis *(See Chapter 5)*	• Females 40 to 60 years old

Most of these disorders can manifest systemically. Their origins are obscure, their courses uncertain, and their cures still undiscovered. Physicians find them all difficult to manage and cannot predict which of their patients will be stricken. Additionally, some patients suffer more than one of the disorders concurrently.

Significance for Clinicians

Although primary care physicians generally diagnose and treat the six rheumatic disorders described in Algorithm 1, afflicted patients may also consult a variety of other clinicians. Therefore, all clinicians, no matter what their specialties, should learn to recognize the signs and symptoms of these disorders because:

1. A patient diagnosed with one or more of the disorders may be taking drugs which could interact adversely with those you are prescribing or intend to prescribe.
2. Each of these patients has a variety of symptoms which you can avoid exacerbating if you understand their significance.
3. A patient with mild signs and symptoms who has not consulted a physician about them can benefit from your explanation of the importance of early treatment.

Autoimmunity

Autoimmunity, which means "self-destruction," is a condition characterized by the body's immune response to its own tissues. Normally, the body's immune system defends against disease by producing antibodies or cytotoxic lymphocytes. These components of the immune system attack invading pathogens and destroy, neutralize, or eliminate them.

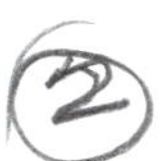

Any part of the body may be altered or damaged by autoimmune reactions.

In some people, however, for unknown reasons, the immune system identifies certain of the body's own components as foreign antigens and attacks them. Normal self-tolerance is lost. Sensitized lymphocytes and autoantibodies gather to destroy tissue cells erroneously identified as invaders, and an inflammatory reaction occurs at the point of attack. Any part of the body may be altered or damaged by autoimmune reactions. If the targets are joints, for example, stiffness, deformities, and hypomobility (limited joint movement) may result.

Autoimmunity is thought to be a significant component of many diseases, especially those affecting connective tissues. Rheumatoid factor (RF), an autoantibody, may be implicated in the progressive inflammation and degeneration caused by rheumatoid arthritis, while numerous circulating autoantibodies, especially antinuclear antibodies (ANAs), may play a major role in the problems engendered by systemic lupus erythematosus.

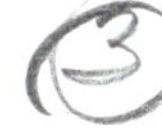

General Clinical Features

The six diseases/syndromes described in Algorithm 1 are usually chronic and often marked by severe flare-ups and spontaneous remissions. Since these disorders have many clinical features in common, it is often difficult to make a specific diagnosis.

Signs and Symptoms

As a first step in determining which of the six disorders they are dealing with, clinicians should assist patients in defining, and differentiating among, the following confusing signs and symptoms:

Arthralgia: Patients may say their arthralgia (joint pain) is throbbing, constant, burning, or excruciating. Clinicians should help patients select more exact terminology, or find an analogy, such as toothache, charley horse, or cramp. The onset and cause of arthralgia differ among the disorders in which it manifests, so clinicians should ask:

1. *When does the pain occur?*
2. *Is its onset sudden or gradual?*
3. *When is it worst?*
4. *How long does the pain last?*
5. *What do you think improves or worsens it?*

Stiffness and hypomobility: Clinicians should pinpoint and inspect the locations of stiffness and hypomobility, then ask:

1. *How long have you had the stiffness?*
2. *What motions does it limit?*
3. *What activities are particularly difficult?*
4. *When does the stiffness occur?* (Motion discomfort occurring after a rest period usually indicates stiffness associated with inflammation, not weakness or fatigue discussed below.)

Weakness and fatigue: To differentiate between weakness and fatigue, clinicians should ask:

1. *Do you have difficulty in gripping objects, chewing, swallowing, standing up, or lifting?* (A positive answer usually indicates weakness, not fatigue.)
2. *Do activity or stress (e.g., exertion, tension, or anxiety) tire you?*
   Do you get some relief from a rest period?
   Do you need more sleep but seldom awaken rested? (Positive answers indicate fatigue, not weakness.)

Appearance

Clinicians should scrutinize the general appearance of patients reporting arthralgia, stiffness, hypomobility, weakness, or fatigue. Inflammatory disorders can produce the classic signs of inflammation: heat, swelling, redness, pain, and loss of function. Free movement of the arms, hands, fingers, and jaw may be interrupted. Posture may become contorted, while the extremities may lose their normal symmetry. Involvement of underlying connective tissue may cause the skin to become tight or drawn, and a rash may appear.

In some cases, the onset is so gradual that patients do not notice their altered appearance. They may not realize that their bites have changed, their walks are different, or their backs are curving. Rarely, however, are they oblivious to pain and a general feeling of malaise and/or disabling fatigue. Alert clinicians will recognize these, and the clinical features described above, as indications of rheumatism.

Roles of Clinicians

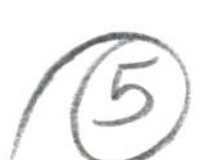

When diagnosing rheumatoid arthritis, fibromyalgia syndrome, systemic lupus erythematosus, Sjögren's syndrome, or systemic sclerosis, most physicians are guided by criteria prepared by committees of the American College of Rheumatology (ACR), formerly the American Rheumatism Association (ARA); for chronic fatigue syndrome (CFS), they use criteria developed by the International CFS Study Group, which includes the Centers for Disease Control and Prevention (CDC). This course provides the criteria for specific diseases in the appropriate chapters.

Patients with manifestations of rheumatism should be given a complete physical examination by a primary care physician. Inspection, palpation, and range of motion provide initial data on patients' skin and their musculoskeletal systems, including the joints, articular cartilage, bone, and skeletal muscle. Laboratory tests should be used to confirm clinical findings. (*For details, see Appendix B.*)

> Primary care physicians can deliver the best care when they have cooperation from all other clinicians.

Primary care physicians can deliver the best care when they have cooperation from all other clinicians (e.g., dentists, dermatologists, ophthalmologists, social workers, etc.). Consultation between primary care physicians and other clinicians is particularly vital before procedures causing trauma or involving incisions, so as to avoid exacerbating patients' problems. All health care workers can offer support and encouragement, monitor patients' progress, report acute episodes, and assist in the long-term management of the disorders.

This coursebook describes the signs and symptoms with which all clinicians should be familiar, in order to provide safe and effective treatment for their patients with rheumatism. For example, if customary examination procedures cause severe pain in an inflamed joint, muscle spasm may follow. However, clinicians who understand rheumatic disorders will take care to support and relax patients' inflamed joints, thereby achieving greater patient cooperation and treatment success.

The text also reports on drugs prescribed for such patients to reduce inflammation, pain, sleep disorders, and other manifestations. All clinicians should determine which prescription and over-the-counter medications their patients are taking, especially before they prescribe others which could precipitate side effects or toxic interactions.

In recent years, new drugs have altered the usual course of the six rheumatic diseases/syndromes discussed in this coursebook and increased patients' life expectancies; most now have normal life spans. However, many of these patients require long-term medical and dental care, and effective delivery of that care requires the cooperation of all clinicians.

Chapter 1 Rheumatoid Arthritis

Rheumatoid arthritis (RA) is a systemic, autoimmune disease in which immune system cells attack articular cells, cartilage, and bone.[1] This process leads to inflammation and damage of synovial joints, most often those of the extremities.

RA characteristics:
- Autoimmunity
- Symmetric, erosive synovitis
- Extraarticular involvement

RA is a chronic disease which, in the majority of cases, develops slowly and insidiously. (*See Articular Manifestations.*) Without treatment, patients with RA are subject to progressive joint destruction, deformities, and disability. Severe extra-articular manifestations can lead to premature death.[2] Early treatment may prevent many of these problems.

History of RA

Symmetric lesions in the skeletons of archaic Indians suggest that RA existed in North America 3,000 years ago.[3] Prior to the 1800s, cases of RA were probably diagnosed as rheumatism, an umbrella term for many types of aches and pains. Subsequently, historic milestones clarified the situation:

1. In 1819, Sir Benjamin C. Brodie (London) clearly described RA, stating that the disease involved synovitis leading to articular cartilage destruction.
2. In the mid-1800s, A. B. Garrod found that most of the articular maladies called rheumatic gout were neither true gout nor true rheumatism; in 1858, he proposed that arthritic or joint disease with some of the external characteristics of rheumatism be called *rheumatoid arthritis.* In 1922, the British Ministry of Health adopted the name, but nosologic disagreement among researchers kept the ARA (now ACR) from accepting the name until 1941.
3. In 1896, Gilbert A. Bannatyne (Bath) published the first radiographs of joints affected by RA.
4. In 1897, Sir George F. Still (London) published the first detailed study of a distinctive, chronic joint disease in children.
5. In 1904, Joel E. Goldthwait (Boston) published the first American classification of the arthritic disorders.[4]

Epidemiology

Between 0.5% and 1.0 % of the world's 5.3 billion population has RA. An elevated prevalence, as high as 6.8%, has been found among certain American Indian tribes, but the disease is rare among some Southeast Asian and Chinese groups.[5]

In the United States, about 2.5 million adults have RA, and an estimated 80,000 to 100,000 children have JRA.

In the United States, about 2.5 million adults have RA;[6] among those >65 years of age, prevalence of the disease can reach >10%.[7] More women than men have clinical symptoms of RA (the female to male ratio is about 2.5 to 1),[7] but the disease affects males more severely.[5] Although the onset of RA can occur at any age, it often affects persons 30 to 60 years old, disabling them during their most productive years and causing major economic losses.[2]

In the United States, an estimated 80,000 to 100,000 children have juvenile RA (JRA). JRA affects more girls than boys; however, the distribution by sex varies among the three subtypes of JRA. (*See Algorithm 3.*)

Etiology and Pathogenesis

The etiology of RA is still unknown. The disease appears to begin with an abnormal immune response to the body's own tissues. Studies suggest that this autoimmune reaction may be induced by articular tissue infection, though joint inflammation appears to continue long after the inciting infection has run its course.[1]

Genetic factors also appear to play a permissive role. RA patients who test positive for rheumatoid factor (RF) often also test positive for specific histocompatibility locus antigens (HLAs), e.g., HLA-DR4. These immune response genes are encoded in the major histocompatibility complex on chromosome 6, and seem to play a role in determining the intensity and duration of an individual's response to antigens.

Development of RA begins with irritation and inflammation of cells of the synovium.

Development of RA begins with irritation and inflammation of microvascular endothelial cells of the synovium (or synovial membrane), which lines the synovia-filled space in which two bones articulate. Chronic synovitis causes hypertrophy of the synovium; an infiltration of cells causes the synovium's superficial cell layer to increase from its normal 1 to 3 cell thickness to a 5 to 10 cell thickness.[7] A thin, healthy synovium in a normal joint is shown in Fig. 1.

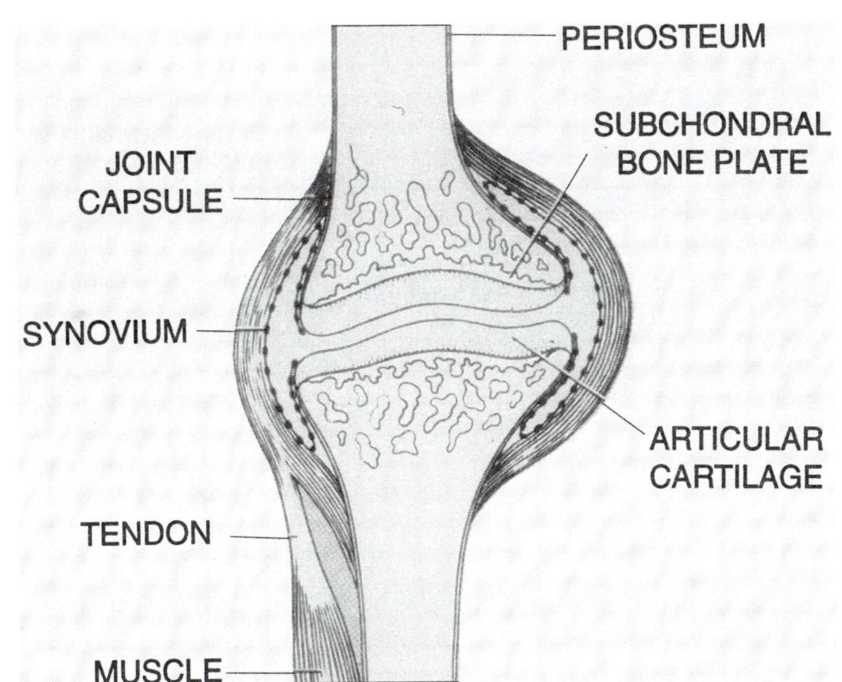

Fig. 1. A normal synovial joint is freely movable within a capsule filled with fluid called synovia. The capsule's surface has a fibrous outer layer and a thin inner layer called the synovium. The articulating surfaces are covered by a smooth layer of cartilage (not by a synovium).

Reprinted from the Clinical Slide Collection on the Rheumatic Diseases, *copyright 1991, 1995. Used by permission of the American College of Rheumatology.*

As the disease progresses, fibroblast-like cells in the synovium's tissues proliferate, forming a pannus (inflamed hyperplastic tissue). This proliferating tissue invades and erodes the periarticular bone and cartilage at the joint margins where synovium and bone are attached. Then, the pannus progressively destroys cartilage over the entire surface of the joint, as well as subchondral bone. When pannus completely fills the once synovia-filled joint space, the joint is ankylosed.[7, 8]

Adult RA Criteria

Many physicians use the ACR's 1987 revised RA classification criteria as the basis for diagnosing the disease in adults; these criteria were established primarily to assure uniformity in research studies of RA.[9 10] As Algorithm 2 shows, a diagnosis of RA is indicated if a patient meets 4 of the 7 criteria.

A majority of patients who fulfill criteria #1 through #5 will probably test RF-positive (criterion #6); however, ≥25% of RA patients test RF-negative, and some patients with other inflammatory conditions (e.g., viral infections, vasculitis, systemic lupus erythematosus, periodontitis) test RF-positive.[11] Therefore, a positive test for RF can support, but not establish, a diagnosis of RA.

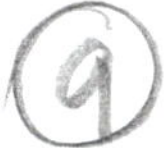

Early in the disease, radiographs have limited diagnostic value, but are useful in establishing a baseline. Once cartilage and bone erosion

Algorithm 2. Adult RA Diagnostic Guide
Presence of 4 of the 7 criteria indicates RA

When evaluating a patient for:	Check for:	Which, if present, fulfills criterion:
Stiffness	Morning stiffness in and around the joints, lasting at least 1 hour before maximal improvement and present for at least 6 weeks	1. Morning stiffness
Soft tissue swelling and synovial effusion	Simultaneous soft tissue swelling or fluid (not bony overgrowth alone) of at least 3 joint areas, lasting for at least 6 weeks and observed by a physician. The bilateral areas to be considered are: **1-2** Proximal interphalangeal (PIP) joints **3-4** Metacarpophalangeal (MCP) joints **5-6** Wrist joints **7-8** Elbow joints **9-10** Knee joints **11-12** Ankle joints **13-14** Metatarsophalangeal (MTP) joints	2. Arthritis of ≥3 joint areas
Swelling of hand joints	At least 1 area swollen (as defined in 2 above) in a PIP, MCP, or wrist joint, for at least 6 weeks	3. Arthritis of hand joints
Symmetric swelling of joints	Simultaneous involvement of the same joint areas (as defined in 2 above) on both sides of the body, for at least 6 weeks. Bilateral involvement of PIPs, MCPs, or MTPs is acceptable without absolute symmetry.	4. Symmetric arthritis
Nodules	Subcutaneous nodules, over bony prominences or extensor surfaces, or in juxtaarticular regions	5. Rheumatoid nodules
Abnormal rheumatoid factor (RF)	Abnormal amounts of serum RF, identified by any method for which the result has been positive in <5% of normal control subjects	6. Serum RF
Bone erosion or decalcification	Changes typical of RA on posteroanterior hand and wrist radiographs, including erosions or unequivocal bony decalcification localized in or most marked adjacent to the involved joints. Osteoarthritis changes alone do not qualify.	7. Radiographic changes

Adapted from Arnett FC, Edworthy SM, Bloch DA, et al. The American Rheumatism Association 1987 revised criteria for the classification of rheumatoid arthritis (Table 5), Arthritis & Rheumatism, 31(3):315-324, *copyright March 1988. Used by permission of Lippincott-Raven Publishers, New York.*

by synovitis begins, radiographic evidence (criterion #7) usually ensues within several months to a year.[10] (*See also Fig. 4.*)

Baseline Evaluation

Not all RA patients have all the classic signs and symptoms of the disease. Therefore, to establish a baseline, primary care physicians take a detailed patient history, do a thorough physical examination, and order specific laboratory tests. Table 1 shows ACR-recommended procedures for a baseline evaluation; these also allow clinicians to rule out other diseases causing arthralgia.[2] (*For characteristics of some of these diseases, see Algorithm 4 at the end of this chapter.*)

Table 1. Baseline Evaluation of RA Patients		
When taking the history, ask patient:	**When examining patient, check for and document:**	**Consider ordering:***
• Describe the degree of your joint pain? • How long does your morning stiffness last? • Which motions does this stiffness limit or prevent? • Do you ever feel fatigued? If so, when?	• Actively inflamed joints • Mechanical joint problems, including: hypomobility; hypermobility; crepitus; malalignment; deformity • Extraarticular manifestations of RA and/or other diseases causing arthralgia	• An arthrocentesis • Blood tests to determine: complete blood count (CBC); erythrocyte sedimentation rate (ESR) or C-reactive protein (CRP); hepatic function; stool guaiac; levels of serum RF, creatinine, and electrolytes • Urinalysis • X-rays of affected joints

* Further explanation of blood and medical tests is given in Appendix B.

Clinical Features of Adult RA

Sixty-five-year-old Charlie steps out of the golf cart, grabs his 7-iron, and walks toward his golf ball lying on the fairway. As he positions himself for the shot, he feels the same stiffness in his swollen ankles that had almost prevented him from getting out of bed a couple of hours earlier. As he swings the club back, then forward and down to make the shot, he feels sharp pain in his wrists. The ball bounces off a tree and lands in a sand trap. Charlie looks at his golf partner and says, "Sorry. I'm through for today. I need to take a good dose of aspirin and see a doctor. Something really bad is happening to my joints." When Charlie's primary care physician hears about the stiffness, swelling, and lingering morning pain, he immediately suspects RA. Laboratory tests and radiographs confirm his suspicions, and he and Charlie formulate a treatment plan.

Articular Manifestations

Clinicians should distinguish between the two categories of RA joint involvement. They are:

1. Potentially reversible, when related to ongoing synovitis. This category's manifestations (e.g., inflammation and stiffness) can be treated pharmacologically and by other nonsurgical methods.

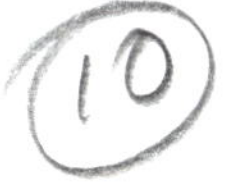

2. Irreversible, when related to structural damage caused by synovitis. This category's manifestations (e.g., cartilage and bone loss) can be treated with physical therapy to control symptoms or, possibly, with reconstructive surgery.[10]

For most RA patients, articular signs and symptoms develop slowly and insidiously over a period of weeks; for about 10% of all RA patients, extensive joint involvement occurs rapidly. About 20% of RA patients have periods of partial or complete remission, followed by involvement of previously unaffected joints.[8]

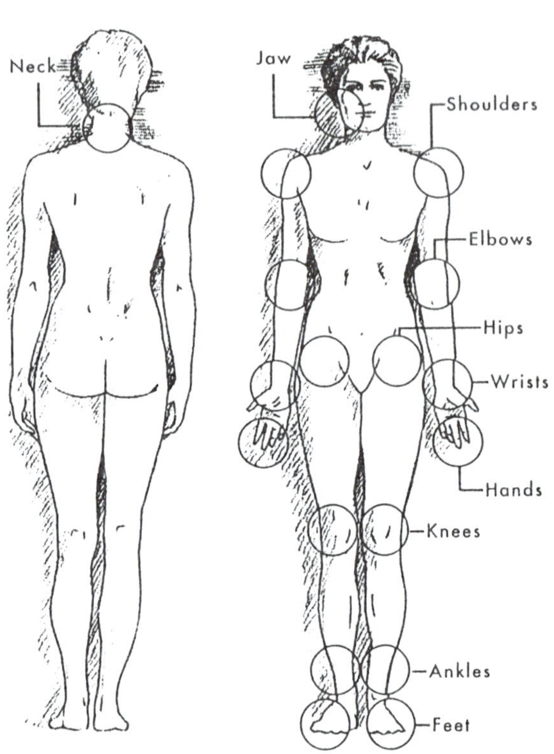

Fig. 2. Joints which rheumatoid arthritis often attacks.
From the brochure Rheumatoid Arthritis, *copyright 1996. Used by permission of the Arthritis Foundation.*

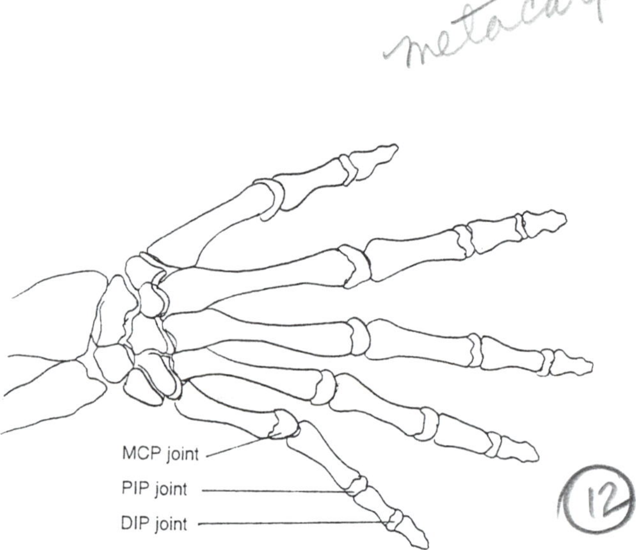

Fig. 3. RA usually affects the MCP and PIP joints, sparing the DIP joint, except in the thumb.

Active synovitis can cause pain and stiffness in any joint, although the thoracic, lumbar, and sacroiliac joints are usually spared.[5] (*See Fig. 2.*) The stiffness, most severe in the morning or after any period of inactivity, is more prolonged than that associated with other arthritic diseases; e.g., the gelling (stiffness after periods of immobility) of osteoarthritis usually lasts only 5 to 10 minutes. RA morning stiffness and pain can persist for ≥1 hour.[10]

Problems which can develop when joints are affected by RA include: (1) loss of motion when patients avoid using a joint because of pain; (2) shortening of muscles adjacent to an inflamed joint; and (3) incongruity of articular surfaces denuded of cartilage. Denuded articular surfaces can be detected in radiographs, or during palpation, which produces a high-pitched, screeching crepitus when the surfaces rub together.[10]

Hand, wrist, and elbow joints: The metacarpophalangeal (MCP) joints, and proximal interphalangeal (PIP) joints in the hands are usually affected by RA. (*See Figs. 3, 4, and 5.*) Unlike osteoarthritis, which often involves distal interphalangeal (DIP) joints, RA does not usually affect the joints closest to the nails, except in the thumbs.[6] Synovitis may cause ulnar deviation at the MCP joints, and swan-neck deformity. RA also attacks elbow and wrist joints. Some RA patients develop carpal tunnel syndrome,[10] in which compression of the median nerve in the wrist causes pain, tingling, and numbness of the thumb and fingers.[12]

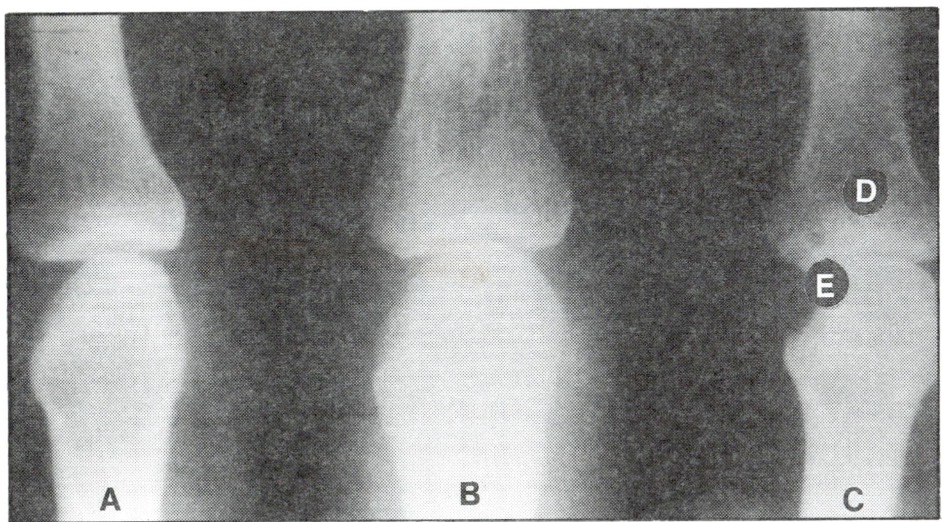

Fig. 4. RA of the Hand. Note the progressive erosion of the MCP joint; in C, loss of bone substance (D) and joint space narrowing (E) are evident.

Reprinted from the Clinical Slide Collection on the Rheumatic Diseases, *copyright 1991, 1995. Used by permission of the American College of Rheumatology.*

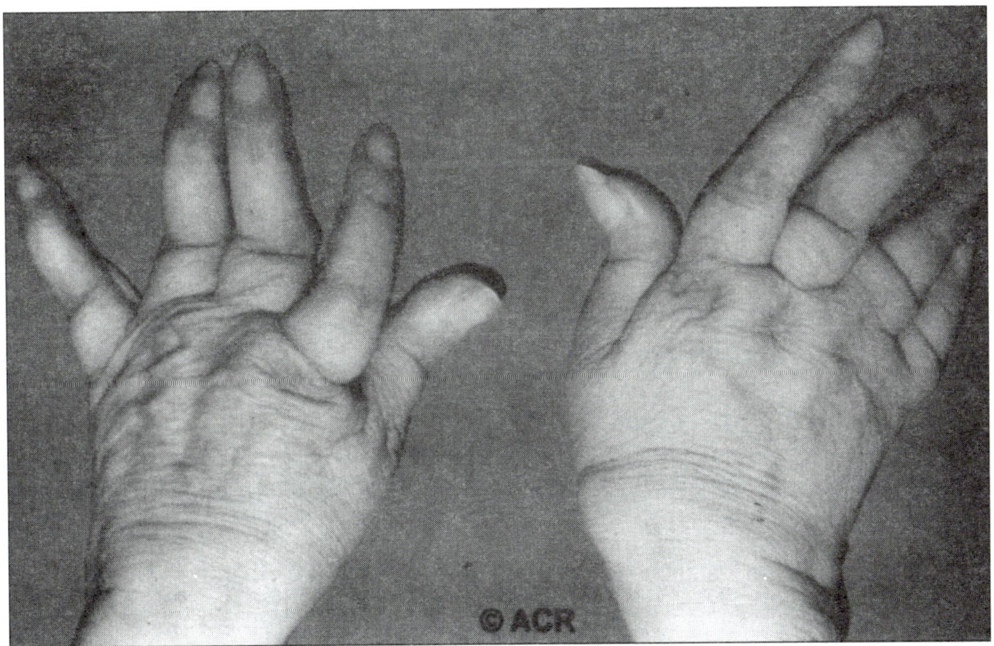

Fig. 5. Wrist and hand deformities caused by chronic RA; severe joint erosion, loss of bone substance, and shortening of digits have led to telescoping and hypermobility of finger joints, and ulnar deviation at the wrist.

Reprinted from the Clinical Slide Collection on the Rheumatic Diseases, *copyright 1991, 1995. Used by permission of the American College of Rheumatology.*

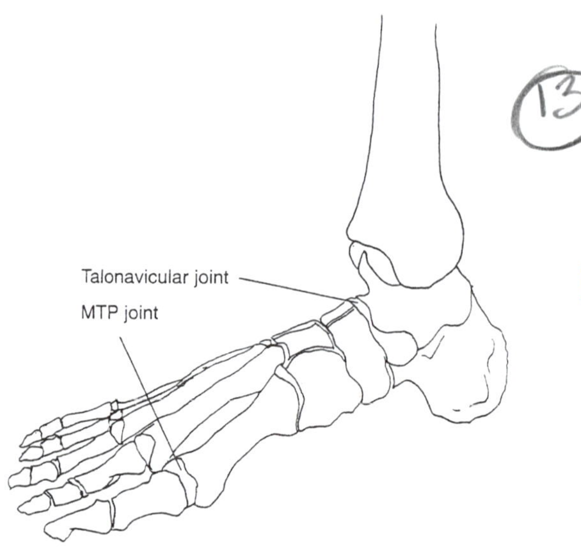

Fig. 6. RA usually affects the MTP and talonavicular joints, causing foot deformities.

Foot, ankle, and knee joints: RA often attacks the metatarsophalangeal (MTP) and talonavicular joints. *(See Fig. 6.)* MTP joint arthritis can lead to: (1) partially dislocated MTP heads, interrupting the normal flow of forces across the joints when a patient stands or walks; (2) cock-up toe deformity; and (3) fibular deviation of toes. (*See color plate E, page 49.*) When the talonavicular joint is inflamed, adjacent muscles go into spasm, making the foot turn outward. Synovitis can also cause tarsal tunnel syndrome, in which compression of the posterior tibial nerve in the ankle produces burning paresthesia on the sole of the foot.[10] Knee thickening, caused by synovial effusion, is detectable on examination, and joint space narrowing is visible in radiographs. (*See Fig. 7.*)

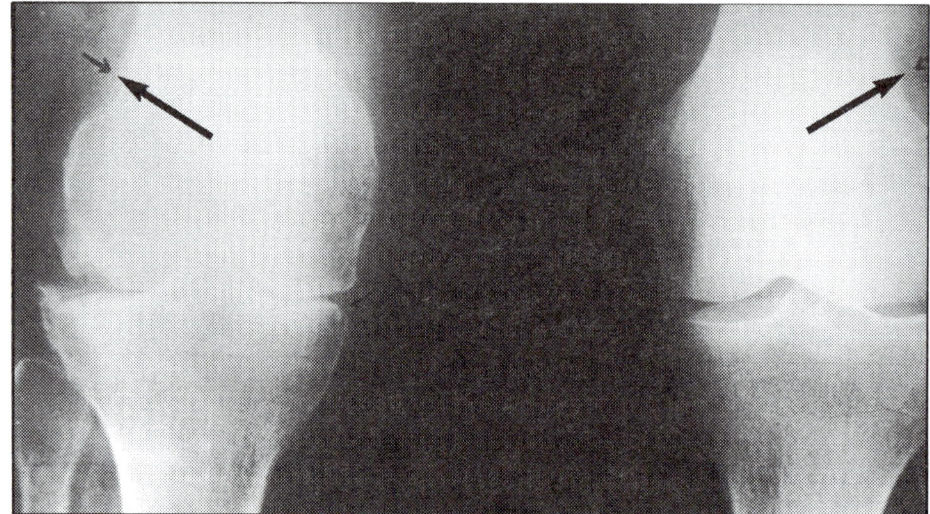

Fig. 7. RA of the Knees. Note the normal joint space in the knee on the right, and the gross but symmetric narrowing of both compartments of the knee on the left; arrows indicate subperiosteal bone formation due to inflammation and remodeling.

Reprinted from the Clinical Slide Collection on the Rheumatic Diseases, *copyright 1991, 1995. Used by permission of the American College of Rheumatology.*

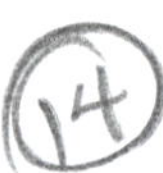

Jaw joints: Whenever a patient complains of temporomandibular joint (TMJ) pain, an alert dentist will check for signs and symptoms of active synovitis in this joint: (1) pain when the patient bites, chews, or yawns; (2) a sudden, distinct change in occlusion; (3) an anterior open bite, which can develop overnight; and/or (4) ankylosis, which can lead to muscle atrophy. (*See also growth retardation, under Juvenile RA.*)

Neck, shoulder, and hip joints: RA frequently causes inflammation of synovial joints in the cervical spine. Initially, the patient has neck stiffness, followed by generalized motion loss.[10] Patients with synovitis in their shoulder joints unconsciously restrict movement of these joints, which often causes ankylosis. When pannus erodes cartilage in the hip joints, symptoms accelerate more rapidly than in nonweight-bearing joints. Patients with RA of the hip joints may feel thigh, groin, low back, or knee pain.[10]

Extraarticular Manifestations

Because RA is a systemic disease, patients often exhibit fatigue, malaise, anemia, and/or generalized musculoskeletal pain. Patients who test RF-positive tend to have extraarticular manifestations (e.g., scleritis, aortitis, pericarditis, pleurisy, and/or pulmonary interstitial fibrosis).[10,14] In addition, the adverse side effects of drugs used to treat RA can manifest as serious systemic complications. (*See Chapter 6.*)

Skin manifestations: With progressive RA, nodules develop in 20% to 30% of patients,[5] usually in subcutaneous tissue overlying bone at pressure areas, especially around the elbows. Fig. 8 shows subcutaneous nodules on the fingers. The nodules, which vary in size from a few millimeters to >5 centimeters,[13] are usually firm, freely-moving, and painless; occasionally, they suppurate, drain, and become subject to secondary infection. Similar nodules can also develop in the synovium, tendons, and viscera (e.g., lungs, pericardium, and myocardium).[5] These

nodules, which are lumps of tissue, differ from the spurs (Bouchard's and Heberden's nodes) which develop at the PIP or DIP joints of patients with osteoarthritis. *(See Algorithm 4.)* Patients with severe, long-standing RA may develop lesions caused by necrotizing vasculitis.[14]

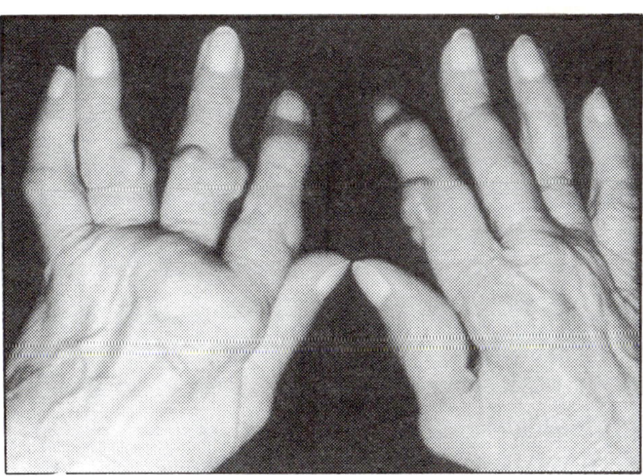

Fig. 8. The subcutaneous nodules seen on the fingers of this RA patient also often occur on the extensor surface of the forearm.

Reprinted from the Clinical Slide Collection on the Rheumatic Diseases, *copyright 1991, 1995. Used by permission of the American College of Rheumatology.*

Some disorders may change RA symptoms; e.g., viral syndromes and nonhemolytic jaundice may induce improvement, while infection, the superimposition of other rheumatic diseases, or a patient's failure to continue therapy may exacerbate RA. Pregnancy may produce either a flare-up of symptoms or improvement of the disease. In most patients, RA waxes and wanes.

Juvenile RA

> *Five-year-old Olivia angrily grabs the sandwich in her lunch box and throws it into the kindergarten classroom wastebasket. Her teacher, who has seen her do this on the previous two days, says: "Olivia, why don't you want to eat your sandwich?" "It hurts my mouth," Olivia whispers. Aware that Olivia has RA in her right knee, the teacher wonders if the disease might be spreading, and mentions the "sandwich problem" to Olivia's mother. A few days later, Olivia's primary care physician refers her to a dentist for x-rays of her temporomandibular joints; the radiographs clearly show TMJ lesions, caused by chronic synovitis, thus explaining the pain Olivia experiences when eating her sandwich. The radiographs also show abnormally small jaws.*

The ACR's revised criteria for diagnosis of JRA, published in 1986,[15] differ from those used for adults and from those used for juveniles in other countries. The ACR diagnostic criteria require that patients:

1. Be <16 years old at onset of the disease
2. Exhibit arthritis in ≥1 joint(s)—defined as swelling or effusion, or the presence of ≥2 of the following: increased heat, tenderness or pain on motion, and/or hypomobility. (The symptoms must be present for ≥6 weeks.)
3. Can be assigned to one of these JRA onset types, following 6 months of active disease:

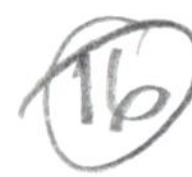

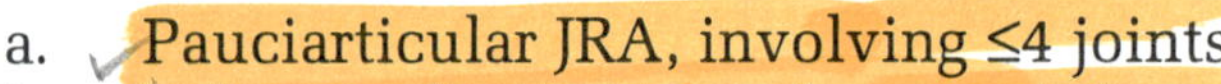

   a. Pauciarticular JRA, involving ≤4 joints
   b. Polyarticular JRA, involving ≥5 joints
   c. Systemic JRA
4. Not have any other rheumatic disease affecting juveniles (e.g., rheumatic fever and infectious arthritis).[15,16]

Algorithm 3 shows signs and symptoms of the three onset types of JRA (pauciarticular, polyarticular, and systemic); subtypes of the pauciarticular and polyarticular onsets have been observed.[16,17,18]

Pauciarticular JRA (up to 50% of children with JRA): Iridocyclitis associated with the early onset pauciarticular subtype is initially asymptomatic in many patients, and an ophthalmologist should admin-

Algorithm 3. Recognizing JRA Onset Types

If a patient exhibits:	Consider:	Which most often affects:
• Synovitis (especially in elbow, wrist, knee, and/or ankle joints); iridocyclitis • Asymmetric synovitis (especially of the hip and other lower extremity joints); sacroiliitis; enthesopathy; iridocyclitis	**Pauciarticular** onset JRA: • Early onset subtype **Pauciarticular** onset JRA: • Late onset subtype	• Females <6 years old • Males >6 years old
• Fever; malaise; anemia • Synovitis (especially in cervical spine joints and symmetric MCP and PIP joints) • Subcutaneous nodules; vasculitis	**Polyarticular** onset JRA: • RF-positive subtype (onset—often ≥8 years old) or • RF-negative subtype (onset—anytime during childhood)	• Both sexes (but female to male ratio is 3:1)
• Spiking fever (temperature of ≥103°), in late afternoon or evening; chills; shaking • Intermittent rash—small, nonpruritic, salmon-pink macules with irregular margins (often on the chest and thighs, but can appear on the face, neck, palms, limbs, and /or soles) • Synovitis (including cervical spine joints); arthralgia • Hepatosplenomegaly; lymphadenopathy; vasculitis; pleurisy; pericarditis	**Systemic** onset JRA	• Both sexes

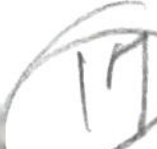

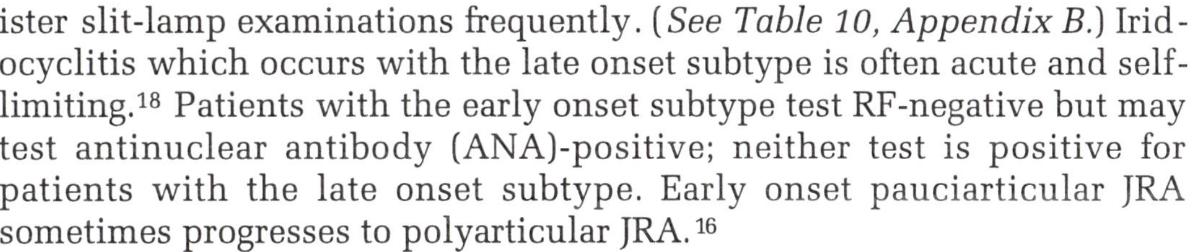

ister slit-lamp examinations frequently. (*See Table 10, Appendix B.*) Iridocyclitis which occurs with the late onset subtype is often acute and self-limiting.[18] Patients with the early onset subtype test RF-negative but may test antinuclear antibody (ANA)-positive; neither test is positive for patients with the late onset subtype. Early onset pauciarticular JRA sometimes progresses to polyarticular JRA.[16]

Polyarticular JRA (about 40% of children with JRA): RF-positive patients, who comprise about 15% to 20% of those with polyarticular onset JRA, have a disease course similar to that of adult onset RA, and are more likely than RF-negative patients to have destructive, disabling arthritis. Up to 33% of patients with polyarticular JRA have delayed development of secondary sexual characteristics and growth retardation.[16] (*See growth retardation below.*)

Systemic JRA (about 10% of children with JRA): In this type of JRA onset, the characteristic rash, often associated with elevated temperature, spreads if rubbed, and fades after a few hours.[19] Joint involvement can also be worse when fever is present, and is sometimes less marked when fever is gone.[18] Chronic polyarthritis often develops weeks to months after onset of systemic signs and symptoms. About 50% of systemic JRA patients eventually have severe, chronic arthritis, with subsidence of extraarticular manifestations, during childhood; others may suffer

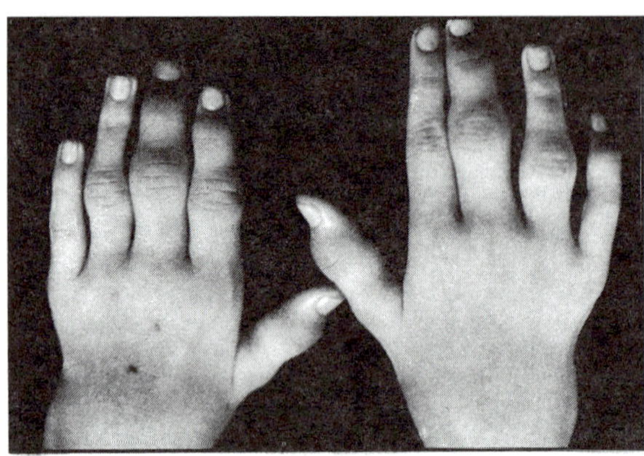

Fig. 9. JRA's effects on a patient's hands. The right second finger has linear overgrowth, and the left fifth finger is foreshortened.

From Jerry C. Jacobs, MD, Pediatric Rheumatology for the Practitioner, *second edition, copyright 1993. Used by permission of Springer-Verlag.*

recurrent systemic problems, as well as chronic arthritis, into adulthood.[16]

Growth retardation: Chronically active JRA can cause overgrowth or undergrowth of bones around inflamed joints (e.g., children with early onset pauciarticular JRA often have unequal leg lengths).[18] Fig. 9 shows bone growth problems in the fingers of a child with JRA. Chronic synovitis of the TMJ can cause micrognathia and a severely receding chin; it can also decrease mandibular function, cause malocclusion, and destroy the mandibular condyle.[20]

RA Treatment

RA treatment is aimed at: (1) reducing synovitis; (2) relieving pain; (3) stopping or slowing joint damage; and (4) improving patients' abilities to function.[6] (*For treatment of patients requiring oral or other invasive procedures, see Endocarditis Prophylaxis, Chapter 6.*)

The ACR reports that patients with active polyarticular, RF-positive RA have a >70% probability of developing joint damage within 2 years of disease onset. Once present, erosive changes are irreversible, so early diagnosis and introduction of appropriate drugs before joint damage occurs are essential to optimal disease management.[2] The primary care clinician, together with the patient, should formulate a treatment plan; the patient is thus informed about:

1. Treatment options and their costs
2. The expected response time
3. Adverse side effects and monitoring requirements of drugs.[2]

Pharmacotherapy

Traditionally, all RA patients were treated for very long periods with nonsteroidal anti-inflammatory drugs (NSAIDs), which reduce joint swelling and pain. When these proved inadequate, as they usually did, to induce remission, so-called "second-line" agents—now called DMARDs—were added. *(See below.)* By then, considerable, irreversible joint damage had often occurred.

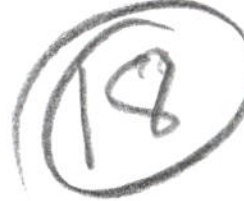

Disease-modifying antirheumatic drugs (DMARDs): Recent studies suggest that early aggressive treatment with DMARDs may alter the course of RA; DMARDs reduce joint damage and preserve joint functioning in some patients.[2,21,22] On the advice of their primary care physicians, most patients still begin treatment with NSAIDs; however, if disease activity persists, they should consult a rheumatologist about starting DMARD therapy. To prevent or slow joint damage, the ACR recommends that DMARD therapy be initiated within 3 months of an established RA diagnosis for patients who, in spite of NSAID treatment, still have:

1. Ongoing arthralgia, or
2. Significant morning stiffness or fatigue, or
3. Active synovitis, or
4. Persistent elevation of the ESR or CRP level.[2] *(See Appendix B.)*

Table 2 shows the approximate length of time various DMARDs require to benefit patients, and some characteristics of each drug.

Table 2. Characteristics of DMARD Therapy

For data on potential adverse side effects of DMARDs, see Chapter 6.

The DMARD:*	Usually benefits patients within:	And is:
Methotrexate (MTX)	1 to 2 months	• Often initially prescribed for patients with severe RA[2] • Expensive and requires intensive patient monitoring for side effects
Hydroxychloroquine (HCQ)	2 to 4 months	• Often initially prescribed for patients with mild RA[2] • Less toxic and less expensive than other DMARDs
Sulfasalazine (SSZ)	1 to 2 months	• Often initially prescribed for patients with mild RA[2] • Particularly effective when used in combination with HCQ and/or MTX
Gold (compound): • Injectablo • Oral	 3 to 6 months 4 to 6 months	• Beneficial for some patients, but often requires 3 to 6 months of administration and frequent patient monitoring for side effects before its effectiveness is determined[6]
Azathioprine (AZA)	2 to 3 months	• Used to suppress overactivity of the immune system when patients are intolerant of gold compounds, HCQ, or MTX[6] • A potent chemotherapeutic agent with potential for significant toxicity
D-penicillamine	3 to 6 months	• Effective in treating vasculitis and neuritis, but can produce the same side effects as gold compounds[6]

* Some researchers prefer the term slow-acting antirheumatic drugs (SAARDs), instead of DMARDs, even though MTX and SSZ can act fairly rapidly.

Of the six currently available DMARDs, methotrexate (MTX) has proved the most predictably beneficial for patients with severe RA; >50% of patients have been able to take MTX >3 years, longer than any other DMARD.[2] However, this drug is expensive, and, because of its adverse side effects, which can manifest as serious complications, MTX requires intensive monitoring, preferably by physicians highly qualified in chemotherapy. *(See Algorithm 11, Chapter 6.)*

Hydroxychloroquine (HCQ) and sulfasalazine (SSZ), less toxic than other DMARDs, are often the initial drugs given to patients with mild RA. Gold compounds administered by intramuscular (I.M.) injection appear to be more efficacious than those taken orally.[2] Azathioprine (AZA), an immunosuppressant, is used to inhibit lymphocyte proliferation, and D-penicillamine is useful in treating moderately severe vasculitis when it accompanies arthritis.

Glucocorticoids (systemic corticosteroids): These drugs can benefit patients by minimizing disease activity during the 1- to 6-month period before a DMARD produces its full effect, thereby making it easier for them to participate in routine daily activities as well as exercise programs aimed at restoring lost joint function. Glucocorticoids may be given either:

1. Orally (e.g., ≤7.5 mg prednisone daily), which appears to slow the rate of joint damage, or
2. Via intraarticular injections (no more than once within 3 months), which can reduce symptomatic inflammation of injected joints.[2, 23, 24]

Use of glucocorticoids must be limited to a short course, because the adverse side effects of these drugs can manifest as serious complications.[2] *(See Algorithm 12, Chapter 6.)* Because of their effects on growth, systemic glucocorticoids are contraindicated for children, unless they have systemic or severe polyarticular onset JRA unresponsive to treatment with MTX or gold compounds.[16]

Experimental pharmacotherapy: Other RA treatments are currently being studied in clinical trials; e.g., Moreland et al.[25] found that RA patients given high doses of anti-tumor necrosis factor α (anti-TNF-α) for 3 months had a 61% reduction in the number of swollen or tender joints. Experimental anticytokine therapy relies on continued suppression of the abnormal amounts of TNF-α found in adult RA patients; like all other current RA drug therapies, it is palliative rather than curative.[26]

Monitoring pharmacotherapy: At each patient visit, primary care physicians should assess the activity of the RA, by re-doing the patient history and physical examination. Because a joint examination may not reveal all structural damage, laboratory tests should also be repeated periodically. (*See Table 1.*) If these procedures indicate that patients' RA is in remission, the treatment plan is working; if the disease is active or progressive, physicians should consider changing and/or adding to patients' pharmacotherapy.[2] Close monitoring for the side effects of each drug mentioned in this chapter is essential. (*See Chapter 6.*)

Nondrug Therapy

Despite pharmacotherapy, some RA patients may suffer structural joint damage which severely limits functioning or produces unacceptable pain. These patients may benefit from surgery (e.g., total hip and/or knee arthroplasty), followed by physical and occupational therapy.[2] Other patients can wear splints specifically designed to support inflamed joints, thereby relieving pain.[17]

Most RA patients can benefit from physical therapy and exercise, which: (1) help maintain joint function; (2) help prevent bone decalcification and muscle atrophy and (3) contribute to the patients' independence and overall conditioning. Bicycling and swimming are preferable to high impact exercises such as running or jumping. However, patients should consult their physicians before starting any exercise programs. (*See Exercising Appropriately, Chapter 7.*)

Finally, adequate rest and a regular bedtime, reduction of stress, and proper nutrition are essential for any chronically ill patient. When RA does flare up, a period of bed rest often benefits the patient. Clinicians and patients can contact agencies listed in Appendix A to obtain further information.

Prognosis

Although no absolute predictions may be made about individual patients, the prognosis tends to be worse for patients with high serum RF titer, swelling of >20 joints, extraarticular manifestations, genetic markers, persistently active RA, and/or radiograph evidence of articular cartilage loss or bone erosion.[2,24] Life expectancy for RA patients is 10 to 15 years below the national average (partly because of drug-induced complications).[5]

All clinicians, no matter what their specialties, can support and encourage RA patients by:

1. Urging them to see their physicians regularly
2. Persuading them to continue their pharmacotherapy and physical therapy
3. Helping them to plan simple, nutritious meals
4. Reminding them that exercise helps to keep their joints supple
5. Motivating them to reduce stress in their lives.

Algorithm 4. Ruling Out Certain Arthritis-like Diseases		
If patient exhibits:	**And is:**	**Consider:**
• Arthralgia • Bouchard's nodes at PIP joints • Crepitus • Heberden's nodes at DIP joints • Joint problems: stiffness (relatively short-lived) after rest periods; enlargement; hypomobility • Loss of hip motion; a limp[27,28]	• ≥65 years of age (majority of patients) • Of either sex, but females are twice as likely as men to have osteoarthritis of the knee[27]	Osteoarthritis, characterized by: • Progressive loss of articular cartilage as patients age • Growth of bone and cartilage at joint margins, leading to spurs • Formation of new bone in the subchondral region, leading to sclerosis[27]
• Arthralgia and hypomobility (one or a few joints) • A bite (dog, cat, or human) • Extraarticular infection (e.g., cellulitis; respiratory, urinary, or GI tract infection; hepatitis B; parvovirus) • Fever (shaking chills in 20% of patients)[29,30]	• Any age, but especially <2 or >60 years of age • Immunosuppressed • A patient with a prosthetic joint • An IV drug abuser[29]	Infectious (or septic) arthritis, characterized by: • Rapid and unpredictable onset • Joint damage, functional disability, and mortality—if not diagnosed early • Association with: RA; systemic lupus erythematosus; chronic hepatic disease; diabetes mellitus; malignancy; sickle cell anemia[29]
• Bone pain, particularly of the chest wall or back (66% of patients) • Carpal tunnel syndrome • Arthralgia (symmetric) • Skin nodules (amyloid-containing)[31]	• An adult female, especially ≥70 years of age[31]	Multiple myeloma, characterized by: • Progressive onset • Well-circumscribed lesions in the skull, ribs, sternum, vertebrae, pelvis, or proximal long bones—as seen in radiographs • Amyloid deposits[31]
• Acute, migratory polyarthritis (85% to 95% of patients), with fever (up to 39°C) • Carditis and/or pericarditis • Erythema marginatum on trunk and face and/or subcutaneous nodules on arm extensor surfaces • Myalgia; prostration • Sydenham's chorea[32]	• 5 to 20 years of age (rare in infants and after age 30)[32]	Rheumatic fever, characterized by: • Acute onset, following Group A streptococcal infection • Cardiac involvement (30% to 90% of patients)[32]
• Arthralgia (asymmetric); joint stiffness • Local enthesopathy: uniformly swollen fingers/toes; chronic hindfoot swelling and pain • Low back pain; myalgia • Urethritis; prostatitis; conjunctivitis; uveitis; diarrhea (sometimes bloody)[33]	• Male (rare in women) • A young to middle aged adult • Genetically predisposed (60% to 80% with HLA-B27 gene)[34]	Reiter's syndrome, characterized by: • Acute onset, usually after a GI or genitourinary tract infection • Inflammation of tendinous insertions into bone (enthesitis) • Association with human immunodeficiency virus (HIV) infection • Lesions on glans penis and soles of feet[33]
• Acute anterior uveitis (25% to 30% of patients) • Back stiffness (worsened by inactivity) • Hip and shoulder arthritis (33% of patients) • Lower lumbar pain (often acute) • Sacroiliitis; spondylitis (common)[35]	• A young adult (aged <40 years) • Male (3 times more common in males) • Genetically predisposed (90% with HLA-B27 gene)[34]	Ankylosing spondylitis, characterized by: • Gradual onset • Chronicity • Inflammation • Rare involvement of extremital joints, ascending aorta, or lungs[35]

Chapter Summary

1. Rheumatoid arthritis (RA) is characterized by autoimmunity; symmetric, erosive synovitis; and extraarticular involvement.
2. RA attacks more women than men; onset of the disease can occur at any age, but is more prevalent among persons 30 to 60 years old.
3. Patients are likely to have RA if they fulfill 4 of the 7 ACR criteria, which are: morning stiffness; arthritis of ≥3 joint areas; arthritis of hand joints; symmetric arthritis; rheumatoid nodules; serum RF; and radiographic changes.
4. Because some RA patients do not exhibit all the classic signs and symptoms of the disease, primary care physicians should: (1) take a detailed patient history; (2) do a thorough physical examination; and (3) order specific laboratory tests, if they suspect the diagnosis.
5. RA stiffness, most severe in the morning or after any period of inactivity, is more prolonged than that found in other arthritic diseases.
6. Articular problems caused by RA include: (1) loss of motion if patients avoid using a joint because of pain; (2) shortening of muscles adjacent to an inflamed joint; and (3) incongruity (e.g., rubbing together) of articular surfaces denuded of cartilage.
7. Synovitis can affect synovial joints in the hands (the MCP and PIP joints); in the feet (the talonavicular and MTP joints); in the jaw (the TMJ); and in the elbows, wrists, cervical spine, shoulders, and hips.
8. Because RA is a systemic disease, patients often exhibit fatigue, malaise, anemia, and/or generalized musculoskeletal pain. Other extraarticular manifestations affecting adult patients include rheumatoid nodules, pleurisy, pericarditis, and/or scleritis.
9. All three JRA onset types involve synovitis; however: (1) patients with pauciarticular JRA can also have iridocyclitis; (2) those with polyarticular JRA can also have subcutaneous nodules and vasculitis; and (3) those with systemic JRA also have a characteristic rash, and can develop hepatosplenomegaly, lymphadenopathy, pleurisy, and/or pericarditis.
10. RA treatment is aimed at: (1) reducing synovitis; (2) relieving pain; (3) stopping or slowing joint damage; and (4) improving patients' abilities to function.
11. Early aggressive treatment with DMARDs may alter the course of RA; among DMARDs, methotrexate is the most predictably beneficial for patients with severe RA.
12. Most RA patients can benefit from physical therapy, exercise, and periods of bed rest.

Progress Test A

1. Onset of RA can occur at any age, but it often affects persons _____ to _____ years old.

2. Chronic synovitis causes hypertrophy of the ____________________.

3. A positive test for RF can _______________, but not define, the diagnosis of RA.

4. For most RA patients, articular signs and symptoms develop ____________ and __________________ over a period of weeks.

5. The morning stiffness associated with RA is ___________ ___________________ than that associated with other arthritic diseases.

6. RA does not usually affect the joints closest to the _________, except in the _____________.

7. Signs and symptoms of active synovitis of the TMJ include pain, occlusal change, an anterior open bite, and _________________.

8. Chronically active JRA can cause overgrowth or undergrowth of bones around ________________ _____________.

9. Patients with active polyarticular, RF-positive RA have a high probability of developing joint damage within ___ __________ of disease onset.

10. If RA disease activity persists despite use of ___________, patients should consult a rheumatologist about starting ___________ therapy.

Check your answers against the progress test answers on page 110. The definitions section, which starts on page 111, is helpful for reviewing terminology associated with the six rheumatic diseases/syndromes discussed in this coursebook.

Chapter 2 Chronic Fatigue and Fibromyalgia Syndromes

CFS characteristics:
- Debilitating fatigue
- Generalized achiness
- Impaired cognition

FMS characteristics:
- Severe fatigue
- Sleep impairment
- Widespread and tender point pain

This chapter discusses two forms of rheumatism—chronic fatigue syndrome (CFS) and fibromyalgia syndrome (FMS)—in which neither inflammation nor autoimmunity is evident. Nonetheless, patients with these syndromes complain of stiffness and pain similar to what is reported by patients with RA and other rheumatic diseases. The two syndromes are widespread, potentially disabling, and readily confused with other rheumatic diseases or syndromes. Their precise nature is unclear, and whether they are even discrete disorders remains controversial.

Epidemiology

In general, fatigue is extremely common: >20% of all adults surveyed at U.S. medical clinics describe fatigue as a major problem.[36] Similarly, musculoskeletal pain is one of the leading causes of disability in the United States. Finally, patients with psychiatric conditions such as somatoform disorder or major depression often complain of fatigue or diffuse, dull, persistent pain, and most patients diagnosed with FMS also fulfill criteria for CFS. Much controversy surrounds diagnoses of CFS and FMS because:

1. Fifty to 80% of patients with CFS or FMS have some manifestations of depression
2. Objective findings on physical examination are lacking
3. Confirmatory laboratory tests do not exist
4. There is diagnostic overlap among numerous pain syndromes.

Nonetheless, the epidemiology of CFS and FMS is indeed distinct from that of other types of rheumatism. Therefore, the National Institutes of Health (NIH) and the ACR, among others, have established diagnostic criteria for these disorders, and actively promote research to resolve the thornier controversies.

Chronic Fatigue Syndrome

Thirty-two-year-old Amy's eyes keep closing as she looks at the computer screen and types the report for her boss. She feels exhausted all the time, even though she goes to bed at 7 o'clock each night and sleeps 12 hours. Four months ago, she had consulted her doctor, thinking she had the flu; he prescribed bed rest and lots of fluids. When her nagging fever, joint aches, and headaches hadn't disappeared in a reasonable time, he ordered a battery of tests—all of which proved negative. At that point, he said: "Just take it easy; I'm sure this will all soon pass." "But how can I take it easy?" Amy now asks. "My life is in shambles: I'm so tired at night I can't do anything for my husband and children, and my boss is making comments about my not getting his work done." "I'm sorry, Amy," the doctor replies. "I can't find any organic reason for your symptoms; would you like a referral to a psychiatrist?" Amy consults another doctor, who refers her to a therapist specializing in stress management techniques.

History of CFS

Over the centuries, numerous names have been applied to the combination of severe fatigue and multiple somatic symptoms now known as CFS. Initially, the names were descriptive: febricula, neurasthenia, and myalgic encephalomyelitis. More recently, attempts to ascribe the disorder to a specific etiology led to terms such as hypoglycemia, chronic Epstein-Barr virus (EBV) syndrome, and, currently, chronic fatigue and immune deficiency syndrome (CFIDS). These terms are either overly specific or imply that more is known about the disorder than is the case. The Centers for Disease Control and Prevention (CDC), therefore, prefer the name chronic fatigue syndrome and have developed CFS case-definition criteria to aid research and to assist physicians in diagnosing the syndrome. (*See Table 3.*)

Etiology and Pathogenesis

The cause of CFS is unknown. Fatigue accompanies many, perhaps most, disorders; it is characteristic of various viral syndromes, especially EBV and human herpesvirus 6 (HHV6), and may persist for weeks or months in a significant percentage of patients with any viral infections. Precisely what causes fatigue in even uncomplicated viral infections, and why it becomes persistent and overwhelming in CFS cases, is unknown. Various cell-signaling hormones, known as cytokines, may be involved; e.g., the presence of abnormally high amounts of TNF and interleukins in patients' blood explain some of the lethargy and malaise accompanying many diseases, from cancer to tuberculosis.

CFS Case-Definition

Table 3 shows the 1994 case-definition of CFS developed by CDC researchers and other members of the International CFS Study Group. Although not intended as definitive for physicians' use, the case-definition can be a helpful diagnostic tool. Patients are considered to have CFS if they fulfill the major criteria and have ≥4 of the 8 symptom criteria concurrently. Patients who have clinically evaluated, unexplained chronic fatigue, but who do not meet the CFS criteria, are considered to have idiopathic chronic fatigue.[37]

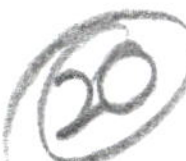

Table 3. Case-Definition of CFS

The major criteria *plus* concurrent occurrence of ≥4 of 8 symptom criteria must be fulfilled.

Criteria	Specifications
Major	Chronic fatigue which is: • Of new or definite onset (not lifelong) and lasts for at least 6 months • Clinically evaluated, unexplained, and persistent or relapsing • Not caused by ongoing exertion • Not substantially alleviated by rest • The cause of a substantial reduction in a patient's previous activity levels
Symptom	Any of the following criteria must have begun at or after onset of debilitating fatigue, and must have persisted or recurred during ≥6 consecutive months of illness: 1. Headaches unlike those normally experienced 2. Myalgia 3. Polyarthralgia (without redness or joint swelling) 4. Prolonged (>24 hrs) postexertional malaise 5. Self-reported impairment in concentration or short-term memory, causing a substantial reduction in a patient's previous activity levels 6. Sleep disorder (insomnia or hypersomnia) 7. Sore throat 8. Tender axillary or cervical lymph nodes

In 1994, the International CFS Study Group also reported conditions which patients can have and still be diagnosed with CFS:

1. Conditions defined primarily by symptoms which cannot be confirmed by laboratory tests (e.g., FMS; anxiety, somatoform, and multiple chemical-sensitivity disorders; depression which is not psychotic or melancholic)
2. Conditions in which alleviation of all symptoms by treatment is verifiable by testing
3. Conditions treated with definitive therapy before chronic symptomatic sequelae develop
4. Any isolated, unexplained test result insufficient to strongly suggest an exclusionary condition.[37] (*See below*)

Conditions excluding patients from a diagnosis of unexplained chronic fatigue are:

1. Those explaining the presence of chronic fatigue (e.g., iatrogenic conditions; narcolepsy; untreated hypothyroidism; sleep apnea)
2. Those whose resolution cannot be documented and whose continued activity might explain chronic fatigue (e.g., unresolved cases of hepatitis B or C; previously treated malignancies)
3. Any current or past diagnosis of depression which is psychotic or melancholic; schizophrenia; dementia; a bipolar disorder; delusional disorder; bulimia or anorexia nervosa
4. Substance or alcohol abuse within 2 years before the onset of chronic fatigue or any time afterward.[37]

Patients, therefore, cannot be diagnosed with CFS if they have any other condition known to cause severe fatigue. For this reason, CFS is often considered a "diagnosis of exclusion," and patients may undergo an enormous battery of tests to exclude everything from malignancies to hormonal abnormalities, acquired immunodeficiency syndrome (AIDS) and toxic exposures, before CFS is diagnosed. Because CFS is so poorly understood, many practitioners believe that it is "only in the mind" and show little sympathy for or interest in its proper identification and treatment. These attitudes are neither appropriate nor helpful.

Table 4 shows the International CFS Study Group guidelines for clinically evaluating patients for CFS.[37] Clinical diagnostic testing for CFS should be done solely to exclude or confirm other possible causes of patients' chronic fatigue.

Clinical Features

The disabling fatigue of CFS, lasting at least 6 months, is usually accompanied by viral-like symptoms; patients often report a generalized achiness and FMS-like tender points.[38] (*See Fig. 10.*) Klonoff reports that, of CFS patients who suffer specific signs and symptoms: 100% have fatigue; 90%, impaired cognition; 85%, joint aches; 80%, myalgia and/or fever; 75%, headaches, weakness, and/or sleep disorders; 50%, enlarged or painful lymph nodes.[39]

CFS Treatment

Physicians experienced in treating CFS, as well as responsive to its sufferers, may initiate appropriate therapy before the diagnosis is absolutely confirmed. In most cases, treatment is safe and does not complicate other conditions; many of the steps benefiting patients with CFS also help those with other causes of fatigue.

Table 4. CFS Clinical Screening and Testing	
Patients should receive:	**Which includes:**
A thorough history-taking	• Circumstances (psychosocial and medical) at the time prolonged or chronic fatigue first began • Descriptions of episodes of medically unexplained symptoms • Current use of drugs (prescription and over-the-counter) and food supplements • Frequency and amounts of alcohol and/or illegal drugs used
A mental status exam	• Identification of abnormalities in personality, intellectual function, memory, or mood
A complete physical exam	• Examination of tender point sites—to rule out FMS (*See Algorithm 5 and Fig. 10.*)
A minimum battery of laboratory tests	• Urinalysis; blood tests to determine: CBC with leukocyte differential; ESR; thyroid function; levels of alanine aminotransferase, albumin, alkaline phosphatase, blood urea nitrogen, calcium, creatinine, electrolytes, glucose, globulin, phosphorus, and total protein *(See also Tables 9 and 10, Appendix B.)*

Therapy for CFS is guided by several general principles:

1. Patients require understanding and emotional support.
2. Patients require relief from their symptoms; since these are so variable, the necessary approach tends to differ from case to case.
3. Since CFS is ultimately neither progressive nor fatal, practitioners must be careful not to expose patients to potential harm from the therapy employed.

On a practical level, treatment begins with various lifestyle changes. Patients are taught to minimize both physical stress caused by strenuous activities and irregular sleep schedules, and emotional stress caused by potentially avoidable situations. Often, these changes may be reinforced by:

1. Cognitive therapy: teaching the patient how inactivity and depression lead to fatigue and physical discomfort
2. Stress management techniques: providing reassurance, improving self-esteem, and using: (a) psychotherapy; (b) biofeedback, to teach relaxation; and (c) acupuncture, which some patients say restores energy.

Certain drugs may further benefit patients. Most prominent among these are tricyclic antidepressants; in low doses, these help relieve the sleep disorders and heightened sensitivity to pain characteristic of CFS. (*For adverse side effects of tricyclics, see Algorithm 14, Chapter 6.*)

Because of the complex nature of CFS, many other types of drugs have also been tested, ranging from intravenous (I.V.) gamma globulin (a blood-derived protein which can cost as much as $100,000 per year and may transmit hepatitis) to antiviral agents and potent pain relievers. None of these has helped CFS sufferers, and, since they expose patients to potential harm without obvious benefit, should be avoided.

Prognosis

At best, CFS tends to be a chronic disorder with remissions and exacerbations. Early treatment with a variety of modalities is most effective. Even without treatment, up to 40% of patients report resolution of their symptoms within 1 year; however, most remain functionally impaired for several years.[37] With CFS, as with other disorders, patience, reassurance, and adherence to the dictum of Hippocrates, "*primum non nocere*" (first do no harm), must be the guides.

Fibromyalgia Syndrome

Forty-year-old Laura sits in her well-cushioned chair, sweat pouring down her face, as she watches the Miami TV weatherman announce that today's temperature will reach 95°F and afternoon showers are expected. She wishes she could turn on her air-conditioner, but, if she does, her persistent pain will only worsen, despite the analgesics she's already taken. The phone rings, and Laura hears the voice of her friend Martha whom she hasn't seen in years. Martha asks: "How have you been?" "Oh, you won't believe what's happened to me; I can't believe it myself," says Laura. "You remember that I used to lead my Girl Scout troop on hikes and camp-outs, and teach classes at the Environmental Center? Well, I had to give it all up! I've got awful pain almost everywhere in my body, I can't get a good night's sleep, and no doctor I've seen can figure out what's wrong with me." Martha says, "I want to help; what can I do for you?" "I don't know," says Laura sadly. "I don't know what anybody can do for me anymore." Fortunately, Martha arranges for Laura to see a doctor who starts her on an exercise program, an analgesic agent to alleviate acute pain, and low doses of amitriptyline to alleviate her insomnia.

History of FMS

Like CFS, fibromyalgia syndrome (FMS) has undergone various changes in name and definition; former names, which have been abandoned, include fibromyosium, muscular rheumatism, and, because it was thought to be caused by inflammation of connective tissue, fibrositis.[40] The complex of symptoms associated with the disorder was described as early as the 17th century.[41] However, the study of FMS was generally neglected until 1977, when Smythe and Moldofsky[42] published a paper proposing diagnostic criteria; this stimulated other researchers to investigate the syndrome.[43]

Etiology and Pathogenesis

Numerous studies have sought a unifying explanation for the signs and symptoms of FMS, and compared various treatment options. When the ACR established criteria defining a relatively uniform patient population, it greatly facilitated clinical trials. Despite this, a fundamental understanding of the disorder remains elusive.

> One theory argues that FMS patients' heightened sensitivity to pain is caused by a disturbance of restorative, delta wave sleep.

One theory about FMS argues that the heightened sensitivity to pain characteristic of the syndrome is caused by a disturbance of restorative, delta wave sleep. This deepest stage of sleep is normally characterized by low-frequency delta waves on an electroencephalogram (EEG), but, in FMS patients, high-frequency alpha wave intrusion occurs.[44]

Research data suggest that certain neurotransmitter, biochemical, and hormonal abnormalities are associated with FMS; these include low levels of serum serotonin, tryptophan, and insulin-like growth factor I; and high levels of cerebrospinal fluid substance P (a neuropeptide associated with pain). However, tests for these abnormalities are neither specific nor sensitive for FMS, so they are not included in clinical screening.[45]

FMS Criteria

Algorithm 5 shows the ACR classification criteria which many physicians use to diagnose FMS (the presence of a second clinical disorder does not exclude the diagnosis). Although FMS shares many characteristics with CFS (including fatigue and achiness), FMS is regarded as a distinct entity on the basis of the 18 tender points which define it. (*See Fig. 10.*)

Palpation of tender points: The 18 tender points are anatomic sites where patients feel pain when 4 kg of pressure is applied; however, palpation of tender points is somewhat subjective (e.g., physicians may press too hard or too gently; patients may have a low pain threshold for palpation, or may be obese). In research studies, a dolorimeter, which controls distribution of pressure, provides more objective results.[44]

Diagnostic laboratory tests: Blood tests should include: (1) a CBC with leukocyte differential; (2) an ESR; (3) a general chemistry panel; and (4) a measurement of thyroxine or thyroid-stimulating hormone. Other tests should be avoided, unless needed to confirm an alternative diagnosis suggested by findings during the history-taking and/or physical examination. Other disorders with similar clinical features include polymyalgia rheumatica, early RA, hypothyroidism, and CFS.[45,46]

Algorithm 5. FMS Diagnostic Guide

Presence of both criteria indicates fibromyalgia

When evaluating a patient for:	Check for:	Which, if present, fulfills criterion:
Widespread pain	Pain which has been present for at least 3 months and includes the following: • Pain in the left side of the body • Pain in the right side of the body • Pain above and below the waist • Axial skeletal pain (cervical spine, anterior chest, thoracic spine, or low back) This definition considers shoulder and buttock pain as pain for each involved site, and "low back" pain as lower segment pain.	1. History of widespread pain
Tender point site pain	Pain, on digital palpation performed with an approximate force of 4 kg, in ≥11 of the following bilateral tender point sites: **1-2** **Occiput**: at the suboccipital muscle insertions **3-4** **Low cervical:** at the anterior aspects of the intertransverse spaces at C5-C7 **5-6** **Trapezius**: at the midpoint of the upper border **7-8** **Supraspinatus**: at origins above the scapula spine near the medial border **9-10** **Second rib:** at the second costochondral junctions, just lateral to the junctions on upper surfaces **11-12** **Lateral epicondyle:** 2 cm distal to the epicondyles **13-14** **Gluteal:** in upper outer quadrants of buttocks in anterior fold of muscle **15-16** **Greater trochanter:** posterior to the trochanteric prominence **17-18** **Knee**: at the medial fat pad proximal to the joint line For a tender point to be considered "positive," the patient must state that the palpation was painful; "tender" is not considered painful.	2. Pain in 11 of 18 tender point sites on digital palpation *(See Fig. 10.)*

Adapted from Wolfe F, Smythe HA, Yunus MB, et al, The American College of Rheumatology 1990 criteria for the classification of fibromyalgia (Table 8), Arthritis & Rheumatism, *33(2):160-172, copyright February 1990. Used by permission of Lippincott-Raven Publishers, New York.*

Clinical Features

Pain (widespread and tender point site), stiffness, fatigue, and a variety of other signs and symptoms characterize FMS.

Pain: Patients with FMS suffer pain similar in magnitude to that suffered by patients with RA; they complain of a generalized achiness which tends to be concentrated axially, and often have diffuse stiffness following inactivity.[44] Although the ACR criteria require that widespread pain be present in all four quadrants of the body, many patients with only unilateral, upper body, or lower body pain have FMS. The chronic pain associated with FMS tends to be migratory and intermittent;[45] its intensity may vary from day to day.[44]

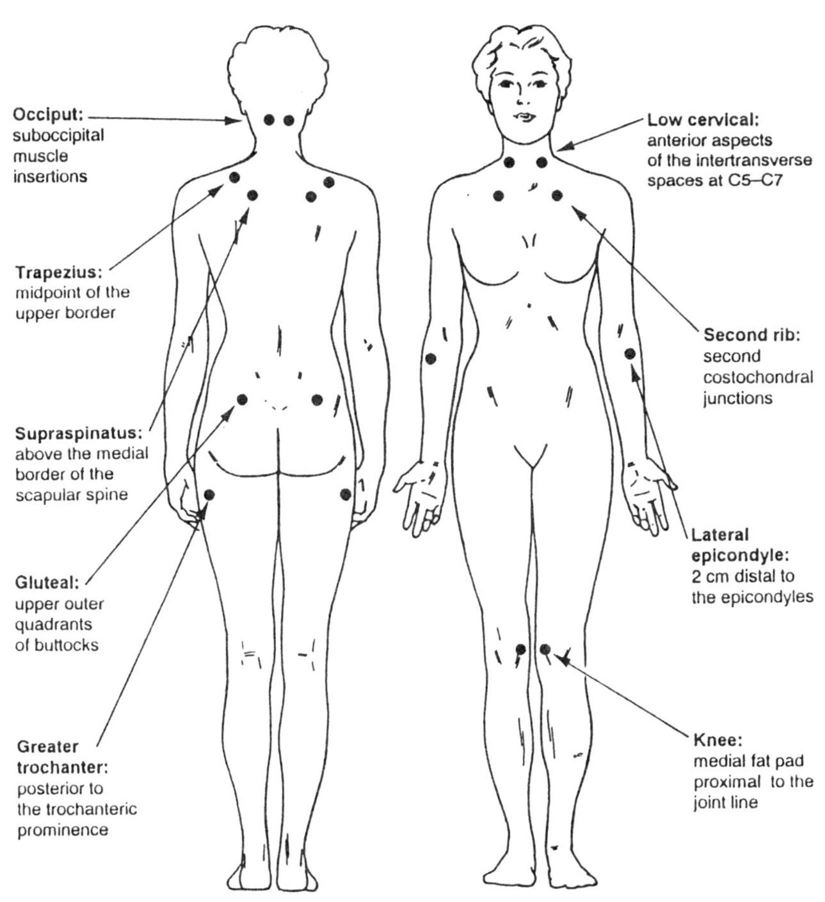

Fig. 10. The 18 tender point sites designated by the ACR for use in diagnosing FMS. *From the* Primer on the Rheumatic Diseases, *tenth edition, copyright 1993. Used by permission of the Arthritis Foundation.*

Fatigue: Many FMS patients report severe fatigue and insomnia. Male patients may have underlying sleep apnea; if spouses report loud snoring and long respiratory pauses, a sleep study may be needed.[44,45] In one study, 70% of the patients with FMS also met the criteria for CFS.[47] *(See Table 3.)*

Visceral and genitourinary manifestations: FMS patients may have increased visceral pain sensitivity. Studies involving randomly selected FMS patients showed a 40% to 70% incidence of esophageal hypomotility (or dysmotility) and a 75% incidence of mitral valve prolapse.[45] In another study, irritable bowel syndrome was reported in up to 50% of patients.[44] FMS patients have an abnormally high incidence of urinary frequency and menstrual pain; some patients may have interstitial cystitis or vulvodynia.[45]

Allergies: Many FMS patients report abnormal sensitivity to perfumes and cigarette smoke, as well as to paint, solvent, and gas fumes that are below established toxic levels. Such reactions, called multiple chemical sensitivities, produce hoarseness, itching or irritated skin, and/or dyspnea.[47] FMS patients also have an abnormally high incidence of lower respiratory symptoms, rhinitis, and nasal congestion.[45]

Neurologic manifestations: FMS patients have an abnormally high incidence of migraine and tension headaches. They may also have nystagmus and difficulties with short-term memory and concentration.[45]

Patients with diffuse paresthesias should be checked for nerve impingement or entrapment, or multiple sclerosis.[46]

FMS Treatment

When a diagnosis of FMS is made, the primary care physician should reassure the patient by explaining that the disorder is not life-threatening; active participation in therapy can improve quality of life.[44,46] With education and reassurance, the physician can alleviate some of the patient's worry and emotional stress.

Treatment of FMS is generally supportive, focusing on increasing a patient's restful, restorative sleep. Algorithm 6 shows various treatments for FMS, all of which may help to alleviate sleep impairment.[44,45,46]

Algorithm 6. Therapy for FMS

For potential adverse side effects of drugs, see Algorithm 14, Chapter 6.

If patient:	Then consider:*	Which:
Has pain amplification and delta wave sleep impairment	• Amitriptyline or doxepin *(tricyclic antidepressants)* • Cyclobenzaprine** *(skeletal muscle relaxant)* *Note: Cyclobenzaprine is structurally related to tricyclics*	• May increase time spent in delta wave sleep, particularly after being taken for 4 to 6 weeks • Can be used in low doses, taken 1 hr before bedtime
Has pain amplification and delta wave sleep impairment—despite low-dose tricyclics	• Alprazolam and zolpidem *(benzodiazepine sedative hypnotics)* • Perphenazine *(phenothiazine antipsychotic)*	• Can be used in low doses to supplement tricyclic antidepressants[45]
Has fatigue as a prominent symptom	• Fluoxetine *(nontricyclic antidepressant)*	• May benefit: (1) patients who have concurrent depression; (2) patients who cannot tolerate tricyclics
Needs pain relief	• Acetaminophen *(analgesic)*	• Should be used only as long as effective, because benefits are marginal
Is suffering depression, stress, and/or insomnia	• Aerobic exercise	• Should begin at a low energy level, and slowly increase • Should involve low-impact aerobic exercises, such as: (1) stationary bicycles or rowing/cross-country skiing machines; (2) water exercise classes • Should be performed 3 times per week, with the goal of increasing the duration to 30 min each time

* Selected brand names are given

** Not in U.S. product labeling for FMS

Continuing studies of FMS treatment are producing interesting results:

1. Goldenberg et al.[48] found that a combination of fluoxetine and amitriptyline produced greater relief of pain and sleep impairment than either medicine alone
2. Russell et al.[49] found that the efficacy of alprazolam was enhanced by the addition of ibuprofen; however, when possible, FMS patients should avoid benzodiazepine sedative-hypnotics, because of their effect on delta wave sleep.

FMS patients should consider avoiding all drugs and participating in nondrug therapy (i.e., psychologic counseling, graded exercise programs, biofeedback, and/or acupuncture). To the extent that these measures restore patients' energy and self-assurance, they are helpful. Finally, an underlying depression contributing to the symptoms of FMS often warrants additional psychiatric intervention.

Prognosis

Although FMS is not usually cured, it is neither progressive nor fatal. The prognosis is better for patients (1) who are young; (2) who have fewer disabling symptoms; (3) who received appropriate medical attention early in the course of the disorder; and (4) who initially had few tender points. However, even patients responding to therapy may report persistent but tolerable pain.[44,46]

Clinicians and patients can contact agencies listed in Appendix A to obtain further information.

Chapter Summary

1. The precise natures of CFS and FMS remain unclear, and their causes unknown.
2. The fact that a patient has certain other conditions does not preclude a diagnosis of CFS; however, patients with conditions known to cause severe fatigue cannot be diagnosed with CFS.
3. Treatment for CFS is safe, and often benefits patients with other causes of fatigue.
4. Both CFS and FMS require that patients' physicians provide them with understanding, support, and relief from their symptoms.
5. Therapy for CFS includes teaching patients to avoid inactivity and depression, and to manage stress. FMS therapy focuses on increasing patients' restful (delta wave) sleep.

Progress Test B

1. Neither ______________________ nor autoimmunity is evident in CFS and FMS.

2. Most patients diagnosed with FMS also fulfill __________________ for CFS.

3. The CFS case-definition can be helpful as a ______________________ __________.

4. Patients cannot be diagnosed with CFS if they have any other condition known to cause ______________ ________________.

5. The disabling fatigue of CFS is usually accompanied by _________________ symptoms.

6. FMS patients' heightened sensitivity to pain may be caused by disturbance of ____________ __________ _____________.

7. The 18 special anatomic sites where FMS patients feel pain when 4 kg of pressure is applied are called ______________ _______________.

8. Male FMS patients may have underlying ____________ __________.

9. Visceral manifestations of FMS include esophageal hypomotility, mitral valve prolapse, and __________________ ______________ syndrome.

10. CFS and FMS patients should limit or avoid ____________________ and participate in ______________ therapy.

Chapter 3 Lupus Erythematosus

Lupus erythematosus (LE) is a general name for several distinct diseases which can be categorized as follows:

1. Systemic LE (SLE), which can involve the skin and virtually any other organ of the body, sometimes producing life-threatening manifestations
2. Chronic discoid LE, characterized by discoid skin lesions which leave scars; about 10% of patients in this category develop SLE after many years
3. Subacute cutaneous LE, characterized by widespread, nonscarring lesions and mild systemic manifestations
4. Drug-induced LE, caused by drugs (e.g., hydralazine, procainamide, chlorpromazine) which induce production of ANAs; the lupus-like syndrome gradually remits with discontinuation of the offending drug(s).[50,51]

This chapter focuses on SLE because about 70% of LE patients have this form of the disease.[52] Antibiotics, glucocorticoids, and improved general medical care have dramatically lengthened the life spans of SLE patients, but no cure has yet been found.

History of LE

In 1845, Ferdinand von Hebra (Vienna) described a butterfly-shaped eruption which appeared on a patient's cheeks and nose. In 1851, Pierre Cazenave (Paris) coined the phrase lupus erythemateux to describe a skin disease which primarily attacked the face, and, in 1872, Moritz Kaposi (Vienna) applied the term lupus erythematosus to cutaneous manifestations in patients he studied.[4,53] There have been other milestones in the study of LE:

1. In 1935, George Baehr and his associates (New York) recognized the exacerbating effect of sunlight on LE patients.
2. In 1948, Malcolm M. Hargraves (Minnesota) described the LE cell found in the bone marrow of several patients with acute SLE. It is

now understood that LE cells are nuclei from fragmented cells coated by ANAs and digested by phagocytic cells.

Epidemiology

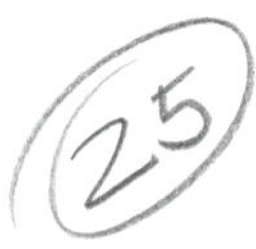

SLE most frequently affects women of child-bearing age, but can also attack men, the elderly, and children (usually newborns and children >4 years of age). During peak incidence of the disease (ages 15 to 40), the female-to-male ratio is at least 5:1.[54,55] African-Americans, Asians, and Native American Indians are more susceptible to SLE than are Whites.[56]

Etiology and Pathogenesis

No single etiologic agent for LE has been identified, but several exogenous factors have been suggested as possible triggers of SLE. (*See Treatment.*) The pathogenesis of SLE is associated with immune dysregulation, which leads to production of abnormal autoantibodies and ineffective clearance of circulating immune complexes. The deposit of these complexes in a variety of tissues activates complement and produces immune-mediated damage.[57]

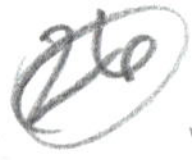

SLE patients tend to produce a variety of autoantibodies; over 95% of patients have serum ANAs, including those targeting the following antigens:

1. Deoxyribonucleic acid (DNA), particularly double-stranded DNA (dsDNA), the form which occurs naturally in nuclei
2. The ribonucleic acid (RNA) protein complexes called Sm, Ro/SS-A, and La/SS-B; the latter two are also found in the serum of patients with Sjögren's syndrome.[54]

Pathologic conditions associated with ANAs include:

1. Active glomerulonephritis—anti-dsDNA is often found in the serum of SLE patients with this serious condition.
2. Neonatal SLE—anti-Ro/SS-A and anti-La/SS-B carried by a pregnant patient can pass through the placenta to a fetus and cause rashes, or heart conduction abnormalities.
3. Abnormal clotting—antiphospholipid antibodies increase the tendency to form thromboses, and may cause strokes, miscarriages, or Raynaud's phenomenon.[54,55]

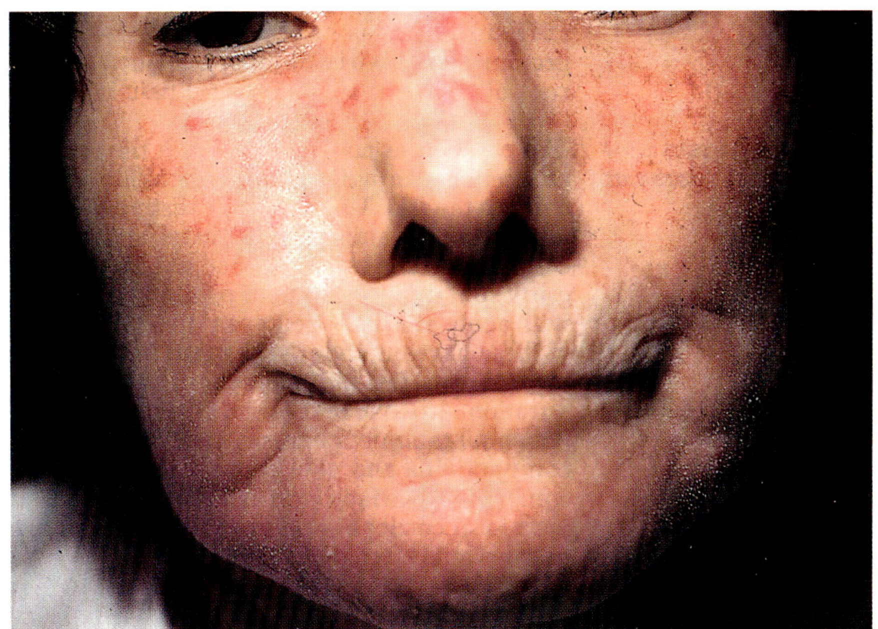

Color Plate

Manifestations of Systemic Lupus Erythematous, Sjögren's Syndrome, Systemic Sclerosis, and Rheumatoid Arthritis

A. Perioral wrinkles of Sjögren's and SSc; note also telangiectasias

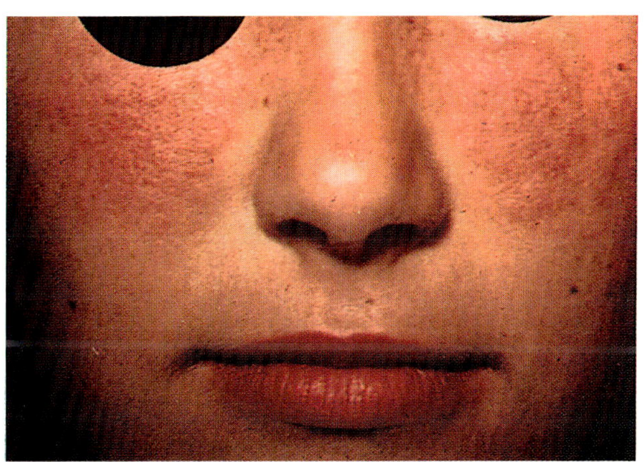

B. Malar rash (butterfly blush) of SLE

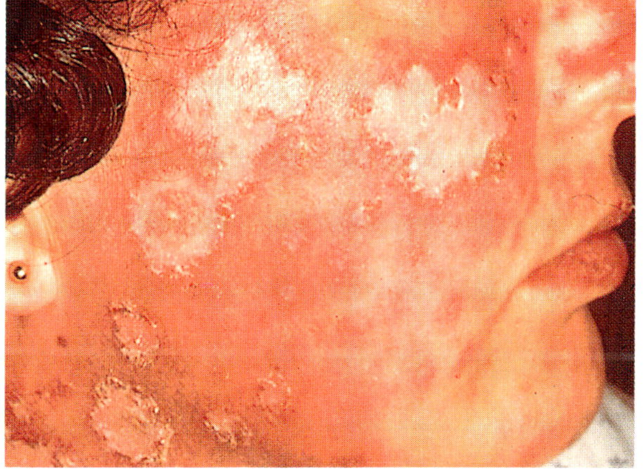

C. Discoid lesions of SLE

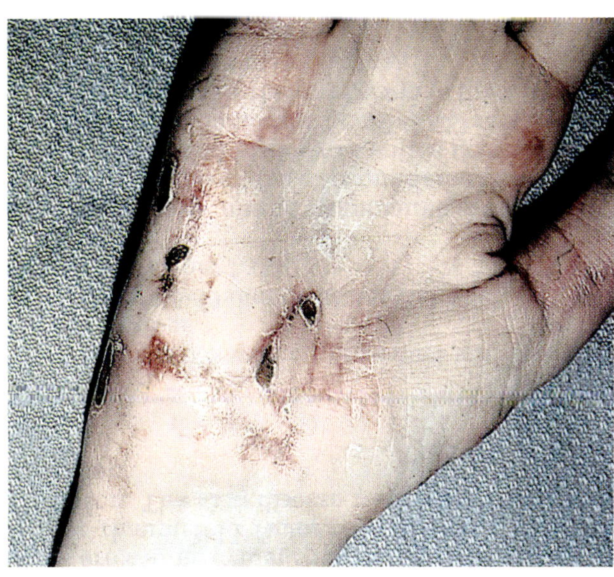

D. Vasculitic skin lesions of SLE

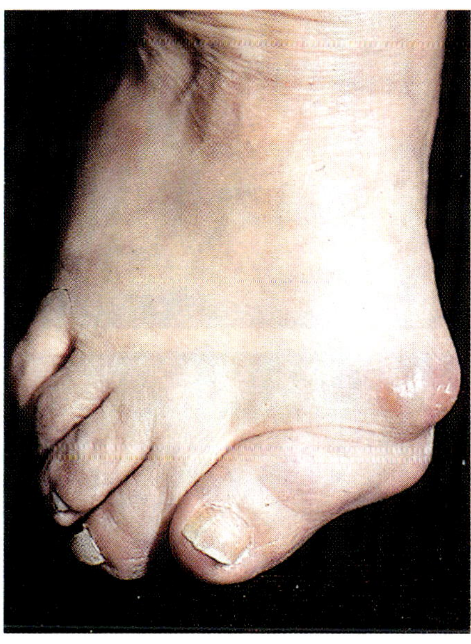

E. Fibular deviation of toes (and resulting bunion at base of first toe) in RA

SLE Criteria

Algorithm 7 shows the ACR's SLE classification criteria, which most physicians use as the basis for diagnosis. Patients are diagnosed with SLE if they meet, over any period, at least 4 of these criteria. The many variations of SLE, in its clinical presentations and intensity of disease course, complicate diagnosis. To confirm a suspected case of SLE, primary care physicians use laboratory tests to check for the presence of one or more of the disorders listed in Algorithm 7.

Hematologic and renal disorders: Diagnostic tests include a CBC; the Coombs' (or antiglobulin) test; urinalysis. *(See Appendix B.)*

Immunologic disorder: Diagnostic blood tests include those for:

1. The LE cell—currently, this labor-intensive test is seldom used,[58] and it is being removed from ACR criteria for classification of SLE. *(See footnote, Algorithm 7.)*
2. Anti-dsDNA and anti-Sm—both are usually found only in the serum of SLE patients; however, levels of anti-dsDNA vary greatly during the course of the disease, which limits the value of this autoantibody as a diagnostic marker.[59] *(See Table 9.)*

3. Antibodies to cardiolipin or other phospholipids may result in a false-positive serologic test for syphilis, detection of a lupus anticoagulant, or artifactual prolongation of in vitro coagulation studies.[59]

Presence of ANAs: Patients with a variety of rheumatic diseases can have a positive fluorescent ANA (FANA) test; therefore, a positive FANA test result should be considered in conjunction with other test results when diagnosing SLE.[59] *(See Table 9.)*

Once a diagnosis is made, clinicians must monitor the disease's fluctuating activity and assess the patient's response to therapy. Both involve laboratory tests, including a CBC, urinalysis, serum complement levels, and anti-dsDNA (the cornerstone of monitoring SLE activity). Levels of anti-dsDNA rise as nephritis worsens, and fall when therapy is effective. In some cases, renal biopsies are necessary (e.g., when serologic data are ambiguous and/or biopsy results would assist in selection of optimum therapy).[59]

Unfortunately, before being diagnosed with SLE, patients often consult several clinicians over many years, with diagnoses of RA, epilepsy, rheumatic fever, nephritis, pleurisy, pericarditis, chronic appendicitis, and/or psychiatric illness. However, when multiple organ systems are affected, and signs and symptoms multiply, classic signs of SLE are more readily recognizable.

Algorithm 7. SLE Diagnostic Guide

Presence of ≥4 criteria, either serially or simultaneously, during any interval of observations, indicates possible SLE when other explanations have been excluded.

When evaluating a patient for:	Check for:	Which, if present fulfills criterion:
Skin manifestations	1. A fixed erythema, flat or raised, over the cheeks, usually sparing the folds of the nose and lips 2. Raised, erythematous, disk-shaped patches, with adherent hard scaling and follicular plugging 3. A rash, or history of a rash, due to an unusual reaction to sun exposure	1. Malar rash 2. Discoid lesion 3. Photosensitivity
Oral signs	4. Oral or nasopharyngeal ulceration	4. Oral ulcers
Musculoskeletal function	5. Nonerosive arthritis involving two or more peripheral joints, with tenderness, swelling, or effusion	5. Arthritis
Cardiopulmonary function	6a. Pleuritis (pleurisy) —the sound of pleural friction rub, evidence of pleural effusion, or a convincing history of pleuritic pain or 6b. Pericarditis—the sound of pericardial rub, evidence of pericardial effusion, or documentation via electrocardiogram (EKG)	6. Serositis
Neurologic function	7a. Seizures not caused by drugs or known metabolic derangements or 7b. Psychosis not caused by drugs or known metabolic derangements	7. Neurologic disorder
Renal function	8a. Persistent proteinuria >0.5g/day or 8b. Cellular casts in the urine, e.g., red cell, granular, tubular, or mixed	8. Renal disorder
Hematologic function	9a. Hemolytic anemia with reticulocytosis or 9b. Leukopenia <4,000/mm^3 total on 2 or more occasions or 9c. Lymphopenia <1,500/mm^3 on 2 or more occasions or 9d. Thrombocytopenia <100,000/mm^3 not caused by drugs	9. Hematologic disorder
Immunologic function	10a. Positive LE cell preparation* or 10b. Anti-dsDNA—antibody to native DNA in abnormal titer or 10c. Anti-Sm—presence of antibody to Sm nuclear antigen or 10d. Antiphospholipid antibody—presence of antibody to negatively-charged membrane phospholipids*	10. Immunologic disorder
Presence of ANAs	11. An abnormal titer of ANA identified by immunofluorescence or an equivalent assay, at any point in time, not caused by drugs which induce lupus syndrome	11. Abnormal ANA titer

Adapted from Tan EM, Cohen AS, Fries JF, et al, The 1982 revised criteria for the classification of systemic lupus erythematosus (Table 37-3), Arthritis & Rheumatism, *25:1271-1277, copyright 1982. Used by permission of Lippincott-Raven Publishers, New York.*

* Item 10a was deleted and item 10d was reworded in 1997 revision—*see Hochberg MC, Updating the ACR revised criteria for the classification of SLE,* Arthritis & Rheumatism, *1997;40(9):1725 (Letter).*

Clinical Features of SLE

Thirty-five-year-old Naomi usually enjoys tending her backyard vegetable garden in Ashville, North Carolina. This summer, for the first time, she's been having trouble keeping up with the weeding and watering. She tires easily, and has remittent fever and aching finger joints. After being in the sun for a couple of hours, she gets a strange-looking rash on her cheeks and the bridge of her nose. Naomi's doctor thinks she might be photosensitive, and tells her to limit her gardening to early morning and late afternoon. "The flu-like symptoms will disappear before you know it," he says. But they don't; they worsen. In the fall, Naomi visits her doctor again, complaining of chest pain and shortness of breath; radiographs show evidence of pericarditis. This condition, combined with Naomi's continuing photosensitivity, causes her doctor to suspect SLE. He runs a battery of tests, including one for anti-dsDNA which proves positive. "Naomi, what you have is a lot more serious than the flu, but, with your help and the latest treatments for SLE, I believe we can control it."

Initial Manifestations

A University of Toronto study of SLE patients indicated that, at onset of the disease, more than 50% of the patients exhibited arthritis and arthralgia, skin lesions, and constitutional signs and symptoms (headache, fever, fatigue, malaise, myalgia, and/or anorexia).[60] Photosensitivity, which affects up to 58% of SLE patients, can cause: (1) abnormally severe sunburn following minimal sun exposure; (2) flare-ups of systemic manifestations; and (3) cutaneous lesions.[51,56]

When SLE is active, there is no uniform pattern of symptoms, and, although some patients have many symptoms, most have only a few which tend to occur repeatedly.[52] In some patients, SLE progresses at a constant rate; in others, it progresses irregularly; in still others, the progression is interrupted by long periods of remission.

Mucocutaneous Manifestations

Cutaneous and mucosal lesions, which develop in over 80% of patients with SLE, are often the first signs causing patients to seek medical attention.[51]

Cutaneous manifestations: Algorithm 8 describes the most common cutaneous manifestations of SLE.[51,56] Although photosensitive patients often suffer acute lupus rashes on various skin areas, the most frequent is the malar rash which usually heals without scarring. *(See color plate B, page 49.)* Discoid lesions, which affect up to 30% of SLE patients, occur on sun-exposed areas of SLE patients' bodies; active peripheral

Algorithm 8. Recognizing SLE Cutaneous Manifestations

If a patient has:	Which:	Then consider:
A symmetric, red-to-violet facial rash shaped like a butterfly (the butterfly's "body" covers the bridge of the nose, while its "wings" spread across the cheeks)	• Develops acutely after sun exposure • Can be a raised or flat erythematous eruption, sparing the nasolabial folds • Does not scar	Acute malar rash *(See color plate B, page 49.)*
A red rash on the dorsum of the hands and between the knuckles (unlike dermatomyositis, which affects skin over the PIP and MCP joints)	• Develops after sun exposure • Can include periungual erythema (indicated by a dark rim around the fingernails)	Acute lupus rash of the hands
A well-circumscribed, red-to-violet, indurated, elevated lesion on the scalp, face, neck, and/or arms. The primary lesion is covered with telangiectasias, atrophic areas, and scale, which, if thick enough, can be lifted to reveal follicular plugs resembling tiny carpet tacks.	• Is chronic • Can vary in characteristics (e.g., plaque may resemble psoriasis; elevation may be minimal) • Often leaves scars; scalp lesions can cause permanent, patchy alopecia	Discoid lesion *(See color plate C, page 49.)*
A blanching, red-to-violet, reticular mottling of the skin; often appears on lower extremities	• May indicate: (1) production of antiphospholipid antibodies; (2) systemic vasculitis	Livedo reticularis

inflammation can cause these lesions to expand, leaving blanched, central scarring.[51] *(See color plate C, page 49.)*

About 50% of SLE patients suffer vascular-related cutaneous lesions, including livedo reticularis, periungual erythema, telangiectasia, and vasculitis. (*See Chapter 5 for telangiectasia; see color plate D, page 49, for vasculitic skin lesions.*) Lesions caused by vasculitis, which develops in up to 20% of SLE patients, include urticaria; painful, punched-out ulcers; and microinfarcts of the fingertips, toes, and nail-fold cuticles. Chilblain lesions afflict about 10% of SLE patients; many patients on long-term steroid therapy develop ecchymoses because of increased skin fragility.[56]

Mucous membrane lesions: These often occur before the patient has other signs of SLE. Oral lesions, which affect about 45% of SLE patients,[61] include:

1. Multiple white plaques with dark, reddish-purple margins[62]
2. Shallow, painless ulcerations of the hard palate[63]
3. Petechiae (*see Fig. 11*) on the buccal mucosa or gingiva, which can develop into shallow, painful ulcers;[61] oral petechiae may indicate thrombocytopenia[63]
4. Discoid erythematous plaques, with central white papules, surrounded by a border of subtle white striae or telangiectatic lesions.[64]

Oral discoid plaques, which usually appear on the buccal mucosa, gingiva, hard palate, and vermilion borders of the lips, can be confused with lichen planus but are distributed less symmetrically.[64] SLE patients can also have candidiasis (caused by corticosteroid use), angular cheilitis, glossitis, mucositis, and periodontitis (particularly when they have xerostomia).[62,63]

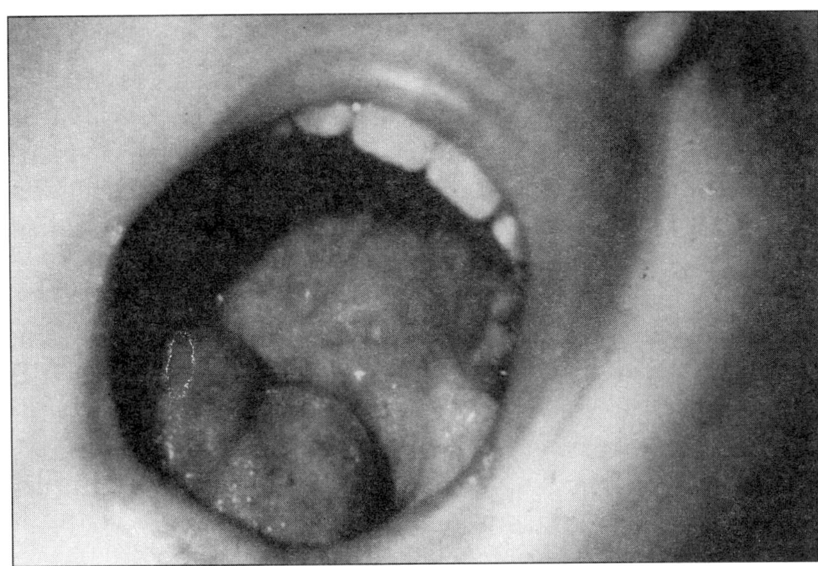

Fig. 11. This patient has scattered vesicles, papules, and petechiae; a vasculitic rash also appears on the tongue.

Reprinted from the Clinical Slide Collection on the Rheumatic Diseases, *copyright 1991, 1995. Used by permission of the American College of Rheumatology.*

When dental clinicians discover a patient has two or more of the oral signs of SLE, or if a single lesion does not respond to standard oral or periodontal therapy, they should refer the patient to an internist or rheumatologist for diagnosis. In general, mucosal lesions represent no danger to the patient, and dental work on SLE patients need not be postponed, except during a lupus flare-up. (*For patients requiring oral or other invasive procedures, see Endocarditis Prophylaxis, Chapter 6.*)

About 20% of SLE patients have nasal ulcers, usually in the lower nasal septum. Ulcers in the upper airway mucosa can cause hoarseness.[56] Although such ulcerations rarely pose a risk to patients, they are a sign of active systemic disease and generally warrant re-evaluation of therapy.

Articular Manifestations

SLE patients often suffer from arthritis, particularly of the wrist, hand, and knee joints. Unlike the severe synovitis affecting many RA patients, that of SLE patients is less acute and does not produce erosions. However, SLE arthritis may nonetheless cause joint deformities (e.g., swan neck deformities; ulnar deviation of the fingers) due to persistent inflammation.[60] In addition, patients with SLE may have overlapping symptoms of other rheumatic diseases (e.g., Sjögren's syndrome and

Raynaud's phenomenon discussed in Chapters 4 and 5, respectively), and these might also affect joints.[52]

Systemic Manifestations

The four most frequent causes of death among SLE patients are infections, glomerulonephritis, seizures, and thrombocytopenia.[51,65] These and other systemic manifestations of SLE are discussed below.

Infections: Clinicians should promptly evaluate unexplained fever. SLE patients are prone to infections resulting from immune system dysfunction or the effects of glucocorticoids and immunosuppressants. Infection should be suspected when a patient not taking these drugs has an elevated white blood cell count, because active SLE seldom causes leukocytosis.[51]

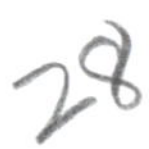

Renal manifestations: Glomerulonephritis, varying in severity and clinical pattern, affects approximately 60% to 75% of SLE patients. Clinicians usually treat active glomerulonephritis aggressively (*see Table 5*); however, when chronic scarring and fibrosis are present, the disease may be irreversible.[59] Symptoms of severe renal problems include hypertension, edema of the legs, extreme fatigue, and anorexia.[52]

Nervous system manifestations: At some time during the course of SLE, approximately 50% of patients suffer nervous system dysfunctions, which can cause severe illness, or even death:

1. Seizures: focal or generalized
2. Central nervous system (CNS) disturbances: organic brain syndrome; coma; stroke; cranial neuropathies (e.g., blindness; nystagmus; tinnitus; facial palsy)
3. Psychiatric disturbances: psychosis; depression
4. Motor and sensory peripheral neuropathies.[59]

Clinicians often have difficulty in determining the causes of nervous system manifestations (e.g., psychosis and depression can be emotional reactions to having SLE, or can result from metabolic anomalies, effects of glucocorticoids, or active lupus).[51]

Hematologic manifestations: Hematologic ailments affecting SLE patients include thrombocytopenia, anemia, lymphopenia, leukopenia, and/or splenomegaly. Refractory thrombocytopenia, a life-threatening condition associated with acute SLE, requires aggressive pharmacotherapy to prevent dangerous hemorrhaging.[60]

Cardiac manifestations: Pericarditis, affecting 20% to 30% of SLE patients, usually causes chest pain and dyspnea, but is sometimes painless without pericardial rub, which can make diagnosis difficult. SLE cardiac manifestations also include myocarditis, coronary artery disease, and endocarditis.[60] (*For patients requiring oral or other invasive procedures, see Endocarditis Prophylaxis, Chapter 6.*)

Pulmonary manifestations: Pleurisy, typically producing small pleural effusions, most often attacks elderly SLE patients or persons with drug-induced LE. Patients with SLE can also develop pneumonitis, pulmonary embolism, pulmonary hemorrhage, or pulmonary hypertension. Before diagnosing pulmonary hemorrhage, clinicians should rule out viral pneumonia; before diagnosing pulmonary hypertension, clinicians should rule out pulmonary emboli, deep venous thrombosis, and intrapulmonary clotting.[60]

Antiphospholipid antibody syndrome (APS): Certain SLE patients have secondary APS, an important cause of hypercoagulability. The presence of circulating antiphospholipid antibodies frequently causes these patients to develop arterial and/or venous thrombosis, strokes, or placental thrombosis which can cause late-pregnancy miscarriages. Less common manifestations associated with the presence of these antibodies include: thrombocytopenia; cardiac valvular vegetations (which can promote bacterial endocarditis); pulmonary hypertension and emboli; and livedo reticularis.[51,66]

Digestive system manifestations: SLE patients often suffer nausea, anorexia, and/or abdominal pain. Although these symptoms usually indicate gastritis or peritonitis, some cases could be caused by pancreatitis or intestinal vasculitis or inflammation. Hepatomegaly may also develop in SLE patients.[60]

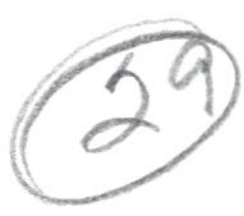

Diffuse alopecia: SLE patients can be affected by two types of diffuse hair problems, both of which, unlike the permanent alopecia secondary to discoid lesions, are usually reversible:

1. The presence (or growth) of abnormally thin, easily fractured hair (called "lupus hair"), usually along the frontal hairline, during exacerbations of SLE
2. Premature hair loss, particularly on the scalp, 3 months after a stressful event (e.g., an SLE flare-up; pregnancy; emotional upset).[56] (*See Fig. 12.*)

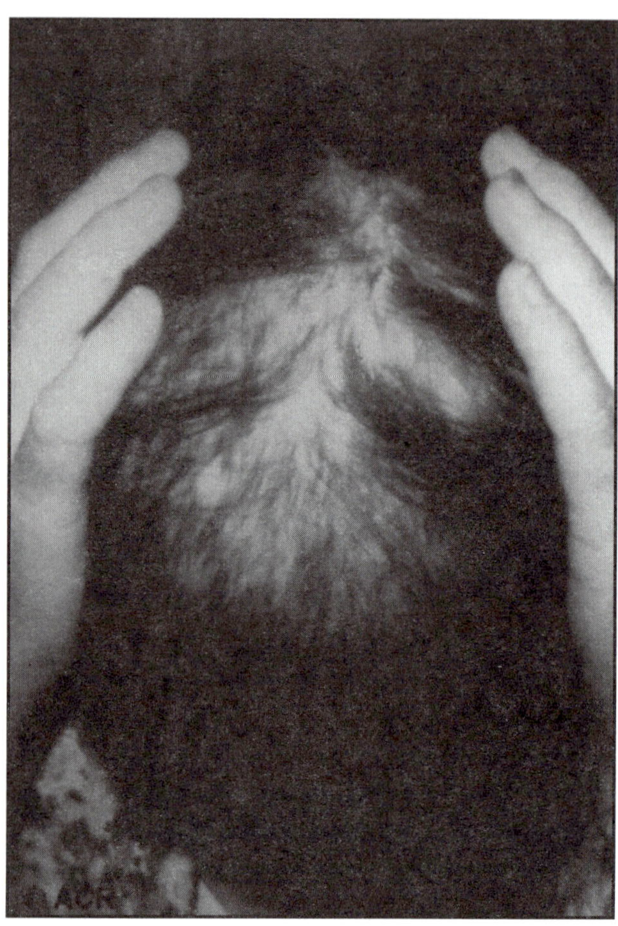

Fig. 12. The diffuse alopecia on the scalp of this SLE patient is caused by an SLE flare-up or another stressful event, not by scarring discoid lesions.

Reprinted from the Clinical Slide Collection on the Rheumatic Diseases, *copyright 1991, 1995. Used by permission of the American College of Rheumatology.*

Treatment

Table 5 shows selected therapies for SLE, which focus on: (1) prevention of acute flare-ups (periods of worsening inflammation); and (2) treatment of secondary disorders.[59,60,67] Pharmacotherapy is used to reduce inflammation and immune system activity, and to alleviate systemic manifestations. However, patients should also balance rest with exercise, and eat properly. (*See Chapter 7.*)

Clinicians should advise patients to avoid potential triggers of an SLE flare-up, including:

1. Sunlight, which can cause inflammation and tissue damage
2. Stress or sleep deprivation, which can stimulate neuroendocrine changes affecting immune cell function.[54]

Table 5. Therapy for SLE

For potential adverse/side effects of drugs, see appropriate algorithms in Chapter 6.

If patient has:	Then consider use of:
Arthritis and arthralgia	• NSAIDs • The antimalarial hydroxychloroquine (HCQ)—if NSAIDs do not give complete relief • Low-dose prednisone—if signs and symptoms persist
Cutaneous manifestations	• Topical corticosteroid—for inflammatory rashes • Intralesional corticosteroid—for discoid LE • Systemic prednisone—for severe discoid LE and cutaneous vasculitis • Dapsone and/or HCQ—for erythematous, inflammatory, and discoid lesions • Sunscreen and protective clothing—to block natural ultraviolet light *Photosensitive patients should also avoid exposure to: (1) sunlight through windows; (2) unshielded, white fluorescent light; (3) artificial ultraviolet light (e.g., halogen lamps; slide projector lights; photocopying machine lights).*
Glomerulonephritis (active proliferative)	• The glucocorticoid prednisone, in conjunction with the immunosuppressant cyclophosphamide (administered pulse I.V. with regular white blood-count monitoring), as recommended by Pisetsky et al.[59] In milder cases, azathioprine might be substituted for cyclophosphamide. *Because guidelines for treating nephritis with these toxic drugs are evolving, clinicians should check the literature for results of ongoing clinical trials.*
Nervous system disturbances	• High-dose methylprednisolone initially, followed by tapering dosages, with or without plasmapheresis—for severe CNS manifestations Exception: heparin initially, followed by oral anticoagulants—for major strokes • Prednisone, plus appropriate anticonvulsant—for seizures • Low to intermediate dose prednisone—for mild neuropsychiatric disorders *Before initiating therapy for neuropsychiatric SLE, clinicians should rule out other causes (e.g., metabolic disturbances; infections; drug toxicities; severe hypertension; uremia).*
Oral lesions	• Hydrogen peroxide or buttermilk gargle, or a steroid-impregnated dental gel—to treat mucous membrane ulcers[61] • Burst therapy, topical clobetasol propionate—to resolve mucosal discoid lesions, followed by maintenance doses of fluocinonide, as recommended by Brown et al.[64] • Thalidomide—to treat refractory cases of mucosal discoid lesions *Patients taking thalidomide must avoid pregnancy.*
Pericarditis; pleurisy	• NSAIDs—for mild symptoms; glucocorticoid—for severe pericarditis or pleurisy *Before initiating treatment, clinicians should rule out drug-caused infections and pulmonary emboli as causes.*
SLE thrombocytopenia	• Danazol, prednisone, and/or immune globulin *Danazol must be used cautiously in patients with renal or hepatic involvement.*

For some patients, elective surgery or pregnancy may trigger or worsen SLE symptoms. Certain drugs cause flare-ups of the disease (e.g., a minority of SLE patients are adversely affected by use of estrogen-containing contraceptives).[51] Before taking any drugs (prescription or over-the-counter), SLE patients should consult with their primary care physicians.[67]

Because their chances of having a miscarriage may be increased, women should be tested for antiphospholipid antibodies if they are pregnant or planning pregnancy. Patients taking drugs which can cross the placenta and adversely affect the fetus should avoid pregnancy. They should use birth control measures because, even though their fertility may be decreased during disease flare-ups, they might still become pregnant. The Arthritis Foundation recommends using a diaphragm (with contraceptive jelly) as the safest contraception method for women with SLE, particularly those adversely affected by estrogen use.[52]

Many local chapters of the Arthritis Foundation offer a 7-week SLE self-help course, which teaches patients to take a more active role in their health care.[52] Clinicians should encourage patients to join a local support group of the Lupus Foundation of America or the Arthritis Foundation. (*See Appendix A.*)

Prognosis

Less than 50 years ago, patients diagnosed with SLE rarely lived more than 2 years. Today, such dismal outcomes are exceptions, thanks to improved treatment of infections and organ system manifestations. Patients who are optimally treated have a 5-year survival rate approaching 93%. Ten-year survival rates are about 75%.[65] Clearly, more advances are needed, but, with appropriate management, the prognosis for patients with SLE continues to improve.

Chapter Summary

1. Lupus erythematosus (LE) can fall into four categories: systemic LE (SLE), chronic discoid LE, subacute cutaneous LE, and drug-induced LE.

2. SLE most frequently affects women of child-bearing age, but can also attack men, the elderly, and children.

3. As a diagnostic marker of SLE, the autoantibody anti-dsDNA has limited value because its levels vary during the course of the disease; however, anti-dsDNA is the cornerstone of monitoring SLE activity.

4. At onset of SLE, more than 50% of patients can exhibit arthritis and arthralgia, skin lesions, and constitutional signs and symptoms; however, when the disease is active, there is no uniform pattern of symptoms.

5. Photosensitive SLE patients often suffer the acute malar rash (butterfly blush), which usually leaves no scar, and discoid lesions, which leave blanched, central scarring.

6. About 50% of SLE patients suffer vascular-related cutaneous lesions, including livedo reticularis, periungual erythema, telangiectasia, and vasculitis.

7. Oral manifestations of SLE can include mucous membrane lesions (e.g., plaques, ulcerations, and petechiae), candidiasis, angular cheilitis, glossitis, mucositis, and periodontitis.

8. Synovitis striking SLE patients is less acute than that affecting many RA patients and does not produce erosions, but it can cause joint deformities.

9. The four most frequent causes of death among SLE patients are infections, glomerulonephritis, seizures, and thrombocytopenia; SLE patients may also suffer hematologic, cardiac, pulmonary, and digestive system manifestations.

10. Two types of diffuse hair problems affecting SLE patients are "lupus hair" and premature hair loss; these are usually reversible, unlike the permanent alopecia secondary to discoid lesions.

11. Therapies for SLE focus on (1) prevention of acute flare-ups; and (2) treatment of secondary disorders.

12. Patients should avoid potential triggers of an SLE flare-up (e.g., sunlight; stress; sleep deprivation).

Progress Test C

1. System lupus erythematous (SLE) can involve the ________ and virtually any other ___________ of the body.

2. SLE patients tend to produce a variety of _______________________.

3. Levels of anti-dsDNA _________ as nephritis worsens, and ________ when therapy is effective.

4. SLE patients often first seek medical attention for ____________________ and _______________ lesions.

5. The acute ____________ rash is shaped like a butterfly, rarely scars, and spares the ____________________ folds.

6. A ______________ lesion often leaves scars and can cause permanent, patchy ___________________.

7. Oral petechiae may indicate ___________________________.

8. SLE arthritis may cause _________ ___________ deformities and ulnar deviation of the fingers.

9. Infections, glomerulonephritis, seizures, and thrombocytopenia are frequent _______________ ___ _____________ for SLE patients.

10. Photosensitive patients should avoid exposure to ______________ and _____________________ ultraviolet light, as well as white fluorescent light.

Chapter 4 Sjögren's Syndrome

Sjögren's characteristics:
- Autoimmunity
- Keratoconjunctivitis sicca
- Nonerosive arthritis with arthralgia
- Xerostomia

Sjögren's syndrome (SS) is a chronic, inflammatory autoimmune disease characterized by diminished exocrine gland secretion (especially from the salivary and lacrimal glands). The disease falls into two categories:

1. Primary SS, when it occurs as an isolated condition
2. Secondary SS, when it occurs concurrently with another autoimmune disorder.[68,69]

History of SS

The first reports of signs and symptoms associated with SS came from European clinicians:

1. In 1892, Mikulica described a male patient with bilateral parotid gland enlargement caused by massive lymphocytic infiltration
2. In 1925, Gougerot reported three patients with salivary and mucous gland secretion insufficiency
3. In 1927, Houwer associated filamentary keratitis with chronic arthritis.[70]

Thon, in 1933, Swedish ophthalmologist Henrik Sjögren reported 19 female patients with keratoconjunctivitis sicca (KCS) and xerostomia; 13 of these patients also had chronic arthritis.[70] Sjögren's (pronounced "show gruns") definitive work led to the disease being named after him.

Epidemiology

SS affects at least 1 million people in the United States. Middle-aged women comprise 90% of the patients with the disease; however, it can afflict both genders and people of all ages and races.[70,71]

Etiology and Pathogenesis

SS is marked by lymphocytic invasion and destruction of exocrine gland tissue (e.g., salivary, lacrimal, and Bartholin's glands, as well as respiratory and GI tract exocrine glands).[70]

The etiology of SS is unknown. Pathogenesis of this syndrome may be related to:

1. Abnormal immunologic responses to unidentified antigens, possibly viral[68]
2. A genetic predisposition to SS (e.g., the presence of HLA-DR-positive epithelial cells in patients' salivary glands, leading to immune recognition and infiltration of glands by lymphocytes).[70]

Patients with SS usually test positive for multiple serum autoantibodies:

1. About 60% to 80% of patients with primary SS test positive for anti-Ro/SS-A and anti-La/SS-B; only 5% to 10% of patients with secondary SS test positive for these autoantibodies.[72]
2. About 90% of SS patients test positive for ANAs[68]
3. About 60% of SS patients test positive for RF. (Patients with SS are at increased risk of developing lymphoma, and the RF may diminish markedly in titer, or disappear, when such malignant transformation occurs.)[68,70]

SS Criteria

Algorithm 9 shows the ACR's SS classification criteria, which most physicians use as the basis for diagnosing primary SS. Patients are diagnosed with the disease if they fulfill 4 of the 6 criteria.

The extent to which clinicians seek evidence of these manifestations of SS varies with different clinical situations. For example, salivary scintigraphy and parotid sialography are difficult and expensive to perform (*see Algorithm 9, criterion 5; Table 10, Appendix B.*) Therefore, dental clinicians should do initial salivary function evaluations during routine examinations:

1. Check to see if the pooled saliva on the floor of the patient's mouth is clear, with a slightly mucoid consistency (patients with xerostomia have foamy saliva which adheres to the palate and buccal mucosa)
2. Determine if a dental instrument or gloved finger slides easily over oral mucosa (these items tend to stick or drag when patients have xerostomia)
3. Determine if saliva flows or a clear droplet forms on the parotid gland orifice when pressure is applied, with a forward movement, to the external skin surface of the parotid gland region (the parotid gland orifice and parotid papillae should first be gauze-dried).[73]

Algorithm 9. Primary Sjögren's Diagnostic Guide Fulfillment of 4 of the 6 criteria indicates primary Sjögren's syndrome		
Ask patient and/or perform test:	**And if:**	**Consider this criterion fulfilled:**
• Have you had daily, persistent, troublesome dry eyes for more than 3 months? • Do you have a recurrent sensation of sand or gravel in the eyes? • Do you use tear substitutes more than 3 times a day?	Patient gives a positive response to at least I of the 3 questions	1. Ocular symptoms (KCS)
• Have you had a daily feeling of dry mouth for more than 3 months? • Have you had recurrent or persistently swollen salivary glands as an adult? • Do you frequently drink liquids to aid in swallowing dry foods?	Patient gives a positive response to at least I of the 3 questions	2. Oral symptoms (xerostomia)
• Schirmer test (≤5 mm in 5 minutes) • Rose bengal score (≥4, according to the van Bijsterveld scoring system) *	Patient has a positive result on at least 1 of the 2 tests	3. Ocular signs (reduced tearing)
• Minor salivary gland biopsy which gives a focus score (focus is an agglomeration of at least 50 mononuclear cells; focus score is the number of foci in 4 mm^2 of glandular tissue)	Patient has a focus score ≥1	4. Histopathologic features of reduced salivary flow
• Salivary scintigraphy • Parotid sialography • Unstimulated salivary flow (≤1.5 mL in 15 minutes)	Patient has a positive result on at least 1 of the 3 tests	5. Salivary gland involvement
• Test for antibodies to Ro/SS-A or La/SS-B antigens • Test for antinuclear antibodies (ANAs) • Test for rheumatoid factor (RF)	Tests indicate presence of at least 1 of the autoantibodies	6. Presence of autoantibodies

* The test involving a rose bengal score is currently seldom used.

Adapted from Vitali C, Bombardieri S, Moutsopoulos HM, et al. Preliminary criteria for the classification of Sjögren's syndrome (Table 4), Arthritis & Rheumatism, *36(3):340-347, copyright March 1993. Used by permission of Lippincott-Raven Publishers, New York.*

If these evaluations initially indicate reduced salivary flow, then they should be repeated at a second appointment after the patient has ingested excess fluids. If reduced flow is confirmed, then a minor salivary gland biopsy should be performed.[73] *(See Algorithm 9, criterion 4.)* This involves sampling of a minor salivary gland in the lower lip or jaw to measure lymphocytic infiltration of acinar tissue.[70] Sjögren's patients usually have >1 focus (a group of >50 mononuclear cells) per 4 mm^2 of sectioned tissue.[68]

Clinicians should also consider testing for reduced tearing and for the presence of autoantibodies listed in Algorithm 9. *(See also Tables 9 and 10, Appendix B.)* In addition, before considering a diagnosis of SS, clinicians should rule out other causes of:

1. Eye dryness (e.g., shrinking of the lacrimal glands accompanying the aging process; use of antihistamines or antidepressants)[72,74]
2. Xerostomia (e.g., use of certain sedatives, antihistamines, antipsychotics, antidepressants, and antireflux drugs with potent anticholinergic effects; effects of radiation therapy for tumors, in which the radiation field includes salivary glands)[75]
3. Parotid gland enlargement (e.g., bacterial or viral sialadenitis; sarcoidosis).[68]

Clinical Features

Charlene, a 45-year-old married woman with two teenaged children, looks at her image in the bathroom mirror. Her eyes are red and itchy; she feels like there's a speck of dirt under her eyelids that won't come out even when she uses eyedrops. Her cheeks are swollen just beneath her ears; her tongue is red and dry; she has a toothache. Lately, she hasn't been able to eat toast or crackers without drinking water after each bite; even then, the food sticks to her mouth. When Charlene visits her doctor, he asks if her eyes feel dry, and if she has to drink water frequently while talking. Her positive answers confirm his suspicion of Sjögren's, so he orders a Schirmer test and some antibody tests. The test results are positive, so he prescribes drugs to relieve Charlene's signs and symptoms, and schedules a follow-up appointment to monitor her parotid gland enlargement. He also tells Charlene, "Patients with Sjögren's often have increased caries because of the lack of saliva, but, with your dentist's close monitoring and your cooperation, these problems can be minimized. Among other things, your dentist can prescribe artificial saliva and topical fluoride treatments, as needed."

Primary SS often involves rapid development of severe KCS and xerostomia, accompanied by parotitis. Primary SS begins as a disease of the exocrine glands, then, 5 to 10 years after its diagnosis, becomes a systemic disease in about 50% of patients. As Fig. 13 shows, SS can affect many body areas. The development of secondary SS in RA patients often involves slowly progressive KCS and xerostomia.[68]

Exocrine Gland Manifestations

Destruction of exocrine gland tissue reduces secretions from these glands, which can cause the problems discussed below.

Ocular manifestations: Patients with KCS often report a sandy or gritty sensation under the eyelids. Other signs and symptoms include itching, burning, and/or red eyes; reduced tearing; photosensitivity; eye fatigue; and excess mucus. Corneal manifestations include ulceration, opacification, vascularization, and, rarely, perforation.[68,70] Patients with

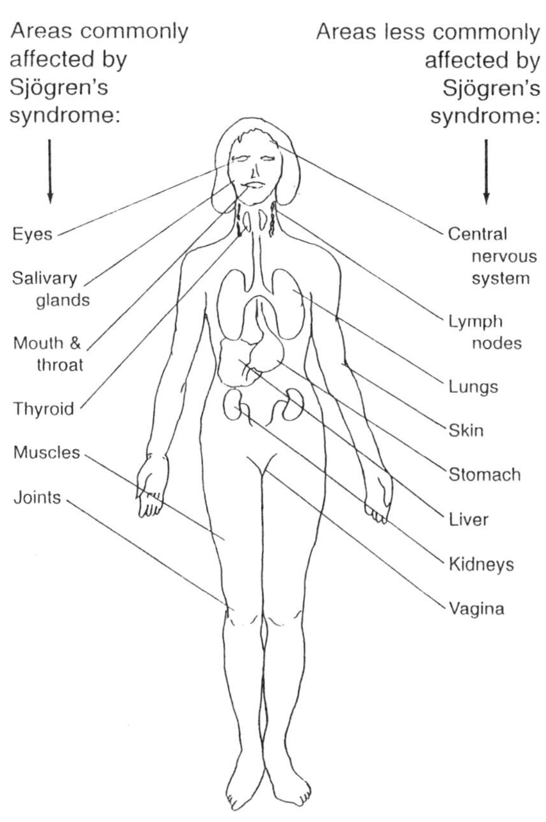

Fig. 13. Areas which Sjögren's can affect.
From the brochure Sjögren's Syndrome, *copyright 1996. Used by permission of the Arthritis Foundation.*

KCS may develop filamentary keratitis, marked by epithelial strands hanging from the cornea.[73]

Oral manifestations: Xerostomia can be continuous or episodic. Patients often report a parched and/or burning sensation in their mouths; adherence of food to buccal surfaces; and problems with chewing, swallowing, and speaking. The tongue can look beefy red, become fissured, and lose its papillae. Patients can develop candidiasis, angular cheilitis, chapped lips, and perioral wrinkles. (*See color plate A, page 49.*) Their taste acuity often decreases, and their caries rate is very high. Parotid gland enlargement, often recurrent, can be accompanied by erythema and fever.[70,76]

Other exocrine glands: Dryness of the nose, larynx, trachea, and/or bronchi, caused by decreased exocrine gland secretion in the respiratory tract, can promote nasal crusting, nosebleed, inflamed sinuses, sore throat, hoarseness, and/or coughing. In some patients, exocrine gland secretion in the GI tract and vagina is diminished. This may lead to abdominal pain, malabsorption, and dyspareunia.[68,70]

Extraglandular Manifestations

Table 6 shows systemic manifestations of primary SS and the approximate percentages of patients they affect. (These manifestations are rare in patients with Sjögren's secondary to RA.) SS patients often suffer fatigue, myalgia, and nonerosive arthritis and arthralgia. Raynaud's phenomenon can precede exocrine gland manifestations by several years. Signs and symptoms of most organ system involvement usually does not appear until 5 to 10 years after primary SS is diagnosed.[68]

Patients with primary SS often have an underactive thyroid; symptoms include cold intolerance, sluggishness, constipation, and deepening of the voice.[72] When persistent, massive, or firm enlargement of major salivary glands is present, clinicians should suspect lymphoma.[68] Most enlarged salivary glands are benign and may exhibit

Table 6. Extraglandular Manifestations of Primary SS		
Involvement of the:	**Affects about:**	**And usually manifests as:**
Joints	60% of SS patients	• Nonerosive arthritis and arthralgia
Fingers and toes	35% of SS patients	• Raynaud's phenomenon (*See Chapter 5.*)
Lungs	14% of SS patients	• Mild lymphoid interstitial disease
Blood vessels	11% of SS patients	• Vasculitis with palpable purpura
Kidneys	9% of SS patients	• Interstitial nephritis with abnormally dilute urine and renal tubular dysfunction (with or without acidosis)
Lymphoid tissues	6% of SS patients	• Lymphoma of major salivary glands

pseudolymphoma (a dense lymphocytic infiltrate), but this condition can progress to malignancy.[76]

Treatment

Primary SS is generally characterized by a rather mild and stable disease course, except for a marked risk of developing malignant lymphoma.[69] Therefore, treatment is usually conservative, except when more aggressive measures are needed to treat pseudolymphoma or malignant lymphoma.[70] Table 7 shows customary therapies for SS, aimed at relieving symptoms and providing fluid or preventing its loss to limit the damaging effects of chronic KCS and xerostomia.[68,70,71,74] Studies indicate that oral, high-dose bromhexine, a gland stimulant, may decrease symptoms of mild to moderate KCS. None of these therapeutic options is curative.

Dental Considerations

Because of diminished salivation, caries is a major problem for SS patients. Meticulous plaque control, with daily flossing and brushing, is mandatory, but patients must not use harsh cleaning agents. Dental clinicians can prescribe for relief of some of these problems. The American Dental Association's (ADA's) *Products of Excellence* lists some of the products available. (*See Clinical Products, Appendix A.*)

Since caries at the gingival interproximal margins can progress quickly in SS patients, they should be monitored with frequent bitewing radiographs. Many dental clinicians advise using a neutral (nonacidic) fluoride gel in a custom carrier for 5 minutes a day, to force the fluoride into the interproximal areas.[76]

Table 7. Therapy for Exocrine Gland Manifestations of SS

If a patient exhibits:	Then consider use of:
Xerostomia	• Water (patient should sip water frequently, particularly with meals); if this fails to relieve dryness, the patient can apply a lubricant (e.g., Vaseline®; mineral oil) to the worst areas • Artificial saliva (e.g., ADA-accepted Saliva Substitute; Salivart® Synthetic Saliva; Xero-Lube Artificial Saliva) • Sugarless gum or candy—to stimulate saliva production
Keratoconjunctivitis sicca (KCS)	• Artificial tear preparations, artificial tear inserts, and ocular lubricants *Patients who repeatedly use artificial tear preparations should consider using preservative-free products. A list of such products is available from the Sjögren's Syndrome Foundation. (See Appendix A.)* • Mucolytic agents • Punctal occlusion—to prevent tears from draining out of the eyes and into the nose • Diving goggles or plastic-wrap occlusion—to prevent tear evaporation at night • Soft contact lenses—to protect the cornea
Dry skin, lips, nostrils, and vaginal mucosa	• Moisturizing lotions—for dry skin • Specifically designed lubricants (not petroleum jelly)—for vaginal dryness • A humidifier

Dental clinicians planning restorative dentistry should consider the risk of recurrent caries. Studies indicate that amalgam may be the best restorative material. Glass ionomer cements and composites are poor restorative choices for an SS patient, because glass ionomer cements lose marginal integrity when dehydrated, and polymerization shrinkage of composite materials causes voids which, in health, are partly offset by the volume of water normally found in saliva.[76] Oral health considerations for patients with rheumatic diseases/syndromes are further discussed in Chapter 7.

Dietary Considerations

SS patients usually have to modify their diets. They should avoid spicy, salty, or acidic foods, and all tobacco items because they irritate the tender tissues. Drinks containing caffeine or alcohol can also exacerbate the condition. Products containing refined carbohydrates promote caries and should be minimized. Foods cooked in broth or gravy are easiest for Sjögren's patients to eat. Examples of nutritious snacks for these patients are:

1. Oat bran cereal, high in water-soluble fiber
2. Endive, watercress, and noncitrus fruit juice combined in a blender to yield a tasty drink high in B and C vitamins
3. Poached fresh fruit, cooled and blended in its own juice.

Since SS patients find chewing difficult, they may suffer from malnutrition. Liquid formula diets (e.g., Ensure®, Sustacal®) and fish oil supplements (e.g., evening-primrose oil, omega 3 fish oils) can provide essential nutrients. Easy-to-eat proteins include soft-cooked eggs, cheese sauce on soft foods, broiled fish, yogurt, and milk. Fruits, vegetables, and whole grains (e.g., oatmeal) provide complex carbohydrates, fiber, vitamins, and minerals. Patients should avoid extremely hot or cold foods, and should gently clean their teeth after each meal. Appropriate foods for patients with rheumatic disorders are further discussed in Chapter 7.

Prognosis

SS can range from a mild malady to a severe generalized affliction. Although periods of remission occur, the disease is most often slowly progressive. However, with careful attention to symptomatic relief, and with close monitoring for development of additional manifestations of autoimmunity, patients can enjoy an excellent quality of life.

All clinicians should be able to recognize the signs and symptoms of SS. Even minor medical and dental procedures must be performed with extreme care. The tissues are tender and easily lacerated. A heavy-handed prophylaxis or a rough examination could cause months of pain or discomfort and exacerbate an underlying rheumatic disease. Even patients in remission require special handling.

Clinicians and patients can contact agencies listed in Appendix A to obtain further information.

Chapter Summary

1. Sjögren's syndrome (SS), characterized by autoimmunity and diminished exocrine gland secretion, primarily affects middle-aged women.

2. Primary SS occurs as an isolated condition; secondary SS occurs concurrently with another autoimmune disorder.

3. Dental clinicians should perform initial salivary function evaluations during routine examinations.

4. Before considering a diagnosis of SS, clinicians should rule out other causes of keratoconjunctivitis sicca (KCS), dry mouth (xerostomia), and parotid gland enlargement.

5. Primary SS often involves rapid development of severe KCS and xerostomia; in secondary SS, KCS and xerostomia progress slowly.

6. The dryness caused by reduction of exocrine gland secretions can cause problems in the eyes, mouth, nose, larynx, trachea, bronchi, GI tract, and vagina.
7. About 60% of SS patients suffer nonerosive arthritis and arthralgia; about 35% suffer Raynaud's phenomenon, which can precede exocrine gland manifestations by several years.
8. Signs and symptoms of most organ system involvement usually does not appear until 5 to 10 years after primary SS is diagnosed.
9. Patients with primary SS often have an underactive thyroid, which can cause cold intolerance, sluggishness, constipation, and deepening of the voice.
10. Customary therapies for SS are aimed at relieving symptoms and providing fluid or preventing its loss to limit the damaging effects of chronic KCS and xerostomia.
11. An increase in caries is the major dental problem for SS patients, necessitating meticulous plaque control and frequent bitewing radiographs.
12. To avoid irritating tender tissues, SS patients should avoid spicy, salty, or acidic foods, and all tobacco items.

Progress Test D

1. Sjögren's syndrome (SS) involves diminished exocrine gland secretion, especially from the ________________ and ________________ glands.

2. Patients with SS usually test positive for ________________ serum autoantibodies.

3. Patients with xerostomia have ____________ ____________ which adheres to the palate and buccal mucosa.

4. Patients with KCS often report a _________ or _________ sensation under the eyelids.

5. Patients with xerostomia often report a ______________ and/or _____________ sensation in their mouths.

6. ________________ ________________ can precede SS exocrine gland manifestations by several years.

7. Oral, high-dose ________________ may decrease symptoms of mild to moderate KCS.

8. When planning restorative dentistry, clinicians should consider the risk of ____________________ ____________.

9. Because they find chewing difficult, SS patients may suffer from ___________________.

10. SS patients' tissues are tender and easily lacerated, so clinicians must perform procedures with _______________ ________.

Chapter 5 Systemic Sclerosis

Systemic sclerosis (SSc), sometimes referred to as "scleroderma," is a generalized disorder characterized by:

1. Fibrosis — excessive synthesis of collagen and its deposit in the skin and other organs causes connective tissues to thicken, harden (or indurate), and lose their ability to function normally.
2. Microvascular injury — the internal lining (or intima) of small arteries thickens, narrowing the lumen and interfering with perfusion of the vascular bed.[77,78]

SSc fibrosis and microvascular injury affect organ systems throughout the body, including the extremities, lungs, GI tract, heart, kidneys, and skin.

Two main SSc subgroups (categorized by the degree of skin and organ involvement), are discussed in this chapter:

1. Limited cutaneous SSc — skin thickening confined to the face, neck, and extremities distal to the elbow and the knee; long-term (years to decades) presence of Raynaud's phenomenon; incidence of pulmonary arterial hypertension and other manifestations late in the disease course
2. Diffuse cutaneous SSc — skin thickening on the trunk, in addition to the face, neck, and distal and proximal extremities; early, extensive organ system involvement (particularly the lungs, kidneys, heart, and GI tract); skin typically becomes puffy or hidebound within 1 year of onset of Raynaud's phenomenon.[77,78,79]

History of SSc

A comment by Hippocrates on a disease marked by "stretched, parched, and hard" skin may be the earliest description of scleroderma. The first clinical report of this skin condition, in 1753, involved a young female patient in Naples, Italy. In the 1840s, other cases were described by British and French physicians; at this time, the disease was thought to involve only the skin, and patients' visceral manifestations were considered separate diseases. However, in 1945, R. H. Goetz suggested that, because of the disease's diffuse nature, "systemic sclerosis" was a more descriptive term than scleroderma.[4,77] Among other historical milestones were the following:

1. In 1862, Maurice Raynaud (Paris) described the circulatory system disease which bears his name; then, in 1899, Jonathan Hutchinson (London) reported a consistent pattern of coexistence of scleroderma and Raynaud's phenomenon.
2. In 1910, Georges Thibierge and Raymond J. Weissenbach (Paris) reported a causal concurrence of scleroderma and calcinosis.
3. In 1942, Prosser Thomas (London) reported a patient with scleroderma who also had calcinosis, Raynaud's phenomenon, esophageal dysfunction, and telangiectasias, and, in 1964, Richard H. Winterbauer (Baltimore, Maryland) suggested that this group of manifestations, with the inclusion of sclerodactyly, be called the CREST syndrome.[4,77]

Epidemiology

Because of the rarity of SSc, epidemiologic data are limited. Females are three to eight times more susceptible than men to idiopathic SSc;[80] however, more males than females may have SSc-like features due to industrial agent exposure (*see below*). Incidence of the disease peaks in persons 40 to 60 years old, but its onset in persons from 5 to 86 years old has been recorded.[77]

Etiology and Pathogenesis

The etiology of SSc is unknown. Its pathogenesis may begin with an endothelial injury, which some researchers hypothesize is caused by an autoimmune response directed against the endothelium.[78] Patients with SSc have disruption of normal endothelial cell functions.[77]

More than 95% of SSc patients test positive for ANAs, including:

1. Anti-RNA polymerases I, II, and III, which are specific for SSc
2. Antitopoisomerase I (formerly Scl-70), found in 30% of patients with diffuse cutaneous SSc and associated with interstitial lung disease
3. Anticentromere, present in 70% to 80% of patients with limited cutaneous SSc.[77,79]

Substances implicated in cases of SSc, or conditions resembling SSc, include:

1. Drugs: appetite suppressants; bleomycin (Blenoxane®); pentazocine (Talwin®); L-tryptophan (*see below*)
2. Industrial agents: Exposure to silica dust, epoxy resin vapors, and hydrocarbons (e.g., benzene; toluene; xylene; vinyl chloride)
3. Breast augmentation chemicals: the presence of silicone in breast implants caused localized skin changes, and has been suspected of causing systemic autoimmune phenomena. Although careful epidemiologic studies have not confirmed an association between silicone breast implants and an increased risk of SSc or other rheumatic diseases, silicone implants are no longer routinely available.[78,81]

Epidemics of environmentally-induced disorders with SSc-like features occurred in:

1. 1981 — contaminated rapeseed oil, sold as cooking oil, produced toxic oil syndrome in nearly 20,000 people in Spain
2. 1989 — a contaminant of the dietary supplement L-tryptophan caused an epidemic of eosinophilic myalgia syndrome in the United States.[78]

The apparent increase in the incidence of SSc over time, as well as the numerous drug- and toxin-induced conditions which resemble SSc, have led many researchers to suspect that SSc is triggered by agents in the environment. To date, neither this theory nor the autoimmune hypothesis has been confirmed.

SSc Criteria

Most clinicians still use the ACR's 1980 preliminary criteria for classification of SSc as a diagnostic guide. As Algorithm 10 shows, a diagnosis of SSc is made if patients exhibit proximal scleroderma (the single major criterion), or 2 of the 3 minor criteria.

The classification criteria, which were not intended for diagnostic use, are less accurate for certain patient groups, including limited cutaneous SSc patients who do not meet the major criterion (proximal scleroderma). When patients appear to fulfill the SSc criteria, primary care physicians use laboratory tests (e.g., for ANAs listed above) to confirm the diagnosis.[79]

Diagnostic tests: Other diagnostic tests for SSc, in addition to those discussed in Algorithm 10, include: (1) nail-fold capillaroscopy, to detect vascular changes; (2) pulmonary function studies, to detect pulmonary involvement; and (3) a barium swallow (radiographic examination of the esophagus), to detect esophageal hypomotility, gastroesophageal reflux, or gastrointestinal dysmotility.[77] *(See also Table 10, Appendix B.)*

Algorithm 10. SSc Diagnostic Guide

Presence of the major criterion, or 2 of the 3 minor criteria, indicates SSc

When evaluating a patient for:	Check for:	Which, if present, fulfills criterion:	Criterion type
Skin manifestations (observation or skin biopsy results)	• Skin tightness, thickening, and nonpitting induration in areas proximal to the metatarsophalangeal or metacarpophalangeal joints, and affecting other parts of the extremities, face, neck, and trunk; the skin changes are usually bilateral, symmetric, and almost always include sclerodactyly (*see below*).	1. Proximal scleroderma	**Major**
Finger and/or toe manifestations	• Skin tightness, thickening, and nonpitting induration limited to the digits • Depressed areas at the tips of digits or loss of digital pad tissue caused by digital ischemia	2a. Sclerodactyly 2b. Digital pitting scars or loss of substance from the finger pad	**Minor** **Minor**
Pulmonary involvement: x-ray or computerized axial tomography (CAT) scan results	• Bilateral reticular pattern of linear or lineonodular densities which are most pronounced in the basilar portions of the lungs and are not caused by another primary lung disease; the densities may resemble diffuse mottling or "honeycombing lung."	3. Bibasilar pulmonary fibrosis	**Minor**

Adapted from Masi AT, Rodnan GP, Medager TA Jr, et al, Preliminary criteria for the classification of systemic sclerosis (scleroderma), (Tables 2 and 9), Arthritis & Rheumatism, *23(5):581-590, copyright May 1980. Used by permission of Lippincott-Raven Publishers, New York.*

Palpation for tendon friction rubs: Primary care physicians should also palpate patients for tendon friction rubs, a sign that fibrosis has affected tendons. If present, tendon friction rubs produce a leathery, rubbing, "squeaking" sensation. These rubs, which often precede widespread skin thickening, are generally found in patients with diffuse cutaneous SSc, particularly at the sites shown in Fig. 14.[82]

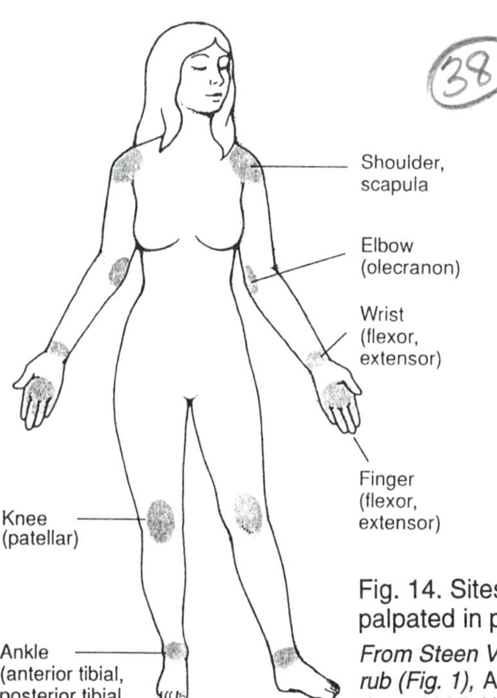

Fig. 14. Sites where tendon friction rubs can usually be palpated in patients with diffuse cutaneous SSc

From Steen VD, Medsger TA Jr, The palpable tendon friction rub (Fig. 1), Arthritis & Rheumatism, *40(6):1147, copyright June 1997. Used by permission of Lippincott-Raven Publishers, New York.*

Clinical Features of Limited Cutaneous SSc

Forty-two-year-old Ramona's boss walks into her office, and she quickly moves her hands from the keyboard to under her desk. Her boss says, "How's the report coming along?" Ramona says, "I'll have it on your desk by 9 a.m. tomorrow," knowing she'll have to work most of the night to finish it because her typing speed has slowed in recent months. For some reason, the skin on her fingers feels tight, making it hard for her to press the keys, and her fingers feel cold even when she's in a warm room. Worried about keeping her job, Ramona visits her doctor. When examining Ramona's face, the doctor sees pinched perioral skin, and asks, " Are you having any problems in opening your mouth?" Ramona says, "Yes. My jaw feels stiff and my tongue hurts when I try to eat or brush my teeth." The doctor says, "I suspect you might have a form of systemic sclerosis. Let me order a few tests to see if other organ systems are involved. If we keep a close watch on any such systems and use appropriate drugs, we can alleviate some of your symptoms. And, with some occupational therapy, we should be able to get your typing back up to speed."

Limited cutaneous SSc, also known as the CREST syndrome, manifests the clinical features listed in the box. The syndrome may be present for years before any organ systems other than the skin are affected by the disorder. The prognosis for limited cutaneous SSc was previously thought to be better than for diffuse cutaneous SSc. It has recently been recognized, however, that a significant percentage of patients with this form of SSc ultimately develop pulmonary arterial hypertension, which has a poor prognosis. If pulmonary function testing reveals a decrease in patients' diffusing capacity, clinicians should consider possible pulmonary arterial hypertension.[77,78]

CREST Syndrome	
C	Calcinosis
R	Raynaud's phenomenon
E	Esophageal hypomotility
S	Sclerodactyly
T	Telangiectasia

Cutaneous involvement usually has three consecutive phases:

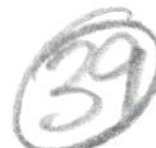

1. Edematous: hands are stiff, with associated puffiness and pruritus (sometimes intense)
2. Indurative: skin is thickened, tight, and shiny, with associated loss of skin folds and changes in pigmentation
3. Atrophic: skin thins because of an ongoing decrease in subcutaneous tissue and dermal perfusion.[77,83]

Calcinosis ("C" of the CREST Syndrome)

Calcinosis usually appears long after other signs and symptoms have emerged. Calcium salts are deposited in the skin, particularly at pressure points (e.g., the finger pads, arm extensor surfaces, and buttocks) and over the joints. Ulceration may allow extrusion of white, gritty material.[77,78] Generally, by the time calcinosis sets in, the other signs and symptoms have led patients to diagnosis and medical care. Figs. 15 and 16 show some of the manifestations of calcinosis.

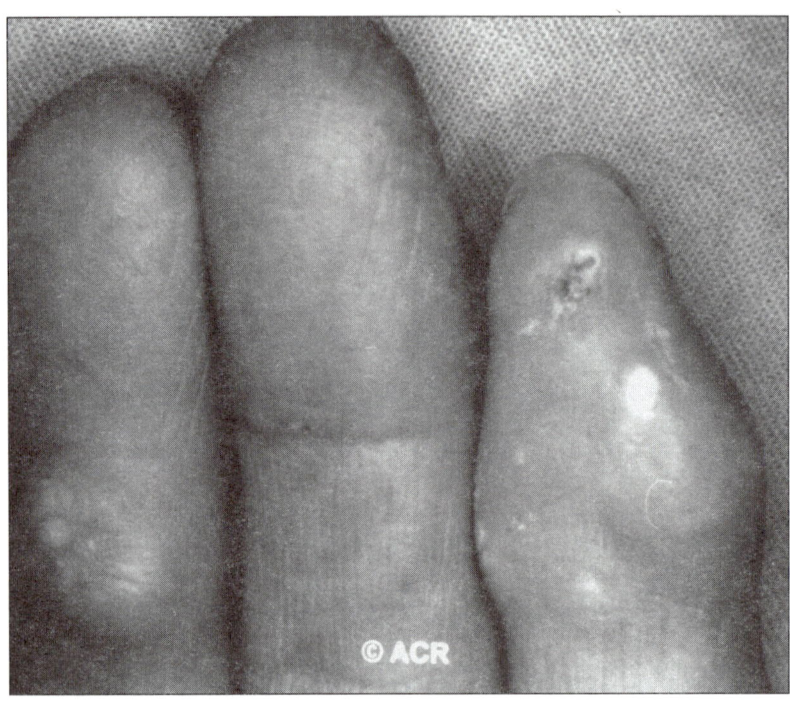

Fig. 15. Signs of calcinosis: irregular, hard nodules, and, at the tip of the index finger, a healing ulcer from which white, gritty material previously extruded.

Reprinted from the Clinical Slide Collection on the Rheumatic Diseases, *copyright 1991, 1995. Used by permission of the American College of Rheumatology.*

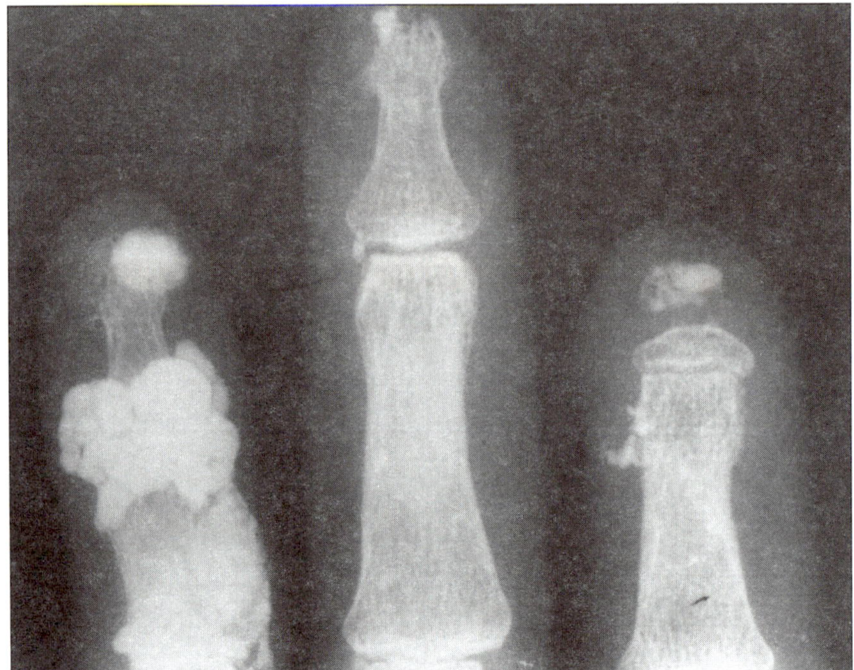

Fig. 16. Extensive calcinosis in an index finger. The x-ray also shows destruction and partial resorption of the tips of the middle and ring fingers.

Reprinted from the Clinical Slide Collection on the Rheumatic Diseases, *copyright 1991, 1995. Used by permission of the American College of Rheumatology.*

Raynaud's Phenomenon ("R" of the CREST Syndrome)

This circulatory system disorder, which affects the fingers and, occasionally, the toes, is the initial complaint of about 70% of SSc patients.[77] When it occurs in association with another disease, it is called secondary Raynaud's phenomenon; when it occurs in isolation, it is called primary Raynaud's phenomenon. The clinical signs are the same in both cases.

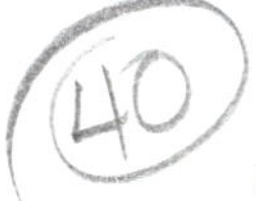

Raynaud's phenomenon, an exaggerated response to cold, is characterized by color changes of the fingers:

1. Paleness (or blanching) occurs when arteriolar spasm causes the small arteries in the fingers to constrict. (*See Fig. 17.*)
2. Blueness (or cyanosis) occurs when blood "pools" in the fingers.
3. Redness (or hyperemia) occurs when vessels open and normal flow is restored.[77,84]

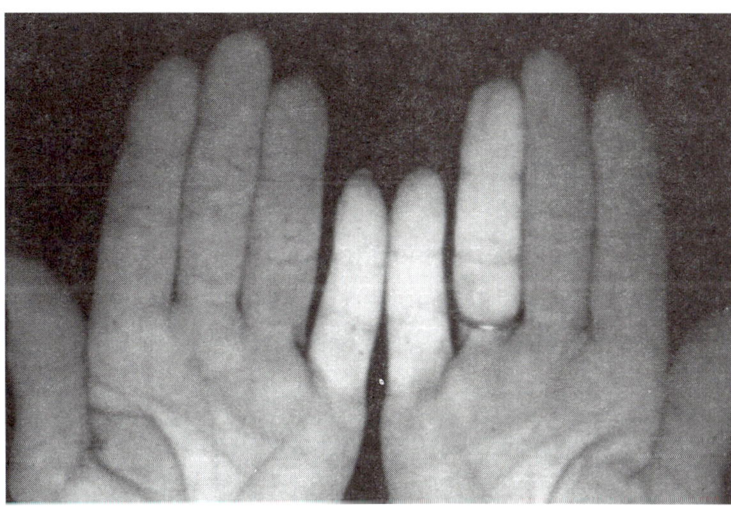

Fig. 17. Blanched fingers characteristic of Raynaud's phenomenon.

Reprinted from the Clinical Slide Collection on the Rheumatic Diseases, *copyright 1991, 1995. Used by permission of the American College of Rheumatology.*

When the fingers are blanched or cyanotic, patients may lose feeling; when hyperemia is involved, patients may suffer pain and tingling. As Raynaud's phenomenon progresses, manifestations of digital ischemia can include:

1. Small, pitted, star-shaped lesions on the fingertips (*See Fig. 18.*)
2. Ulcerations which may become infected
3. Resorption of distal bony tufts, leaving unevenly shortened fingers (*Scc Fig. 19.*)
4. Gangrene of distal digits and autoamputation.[77,85]

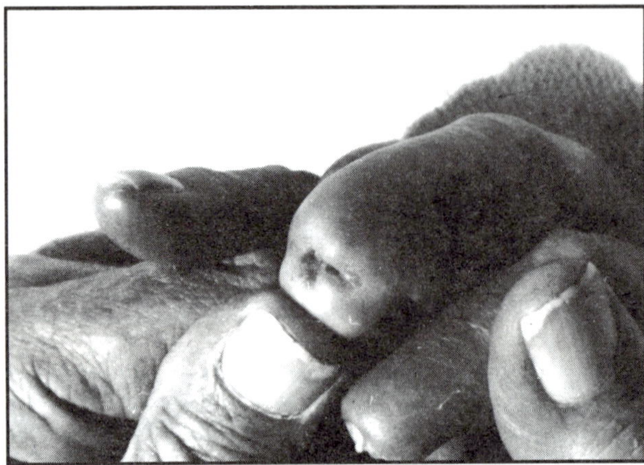

Fig. 18. A star-shaped lesion caused by severe Raynaud's phenomenon.

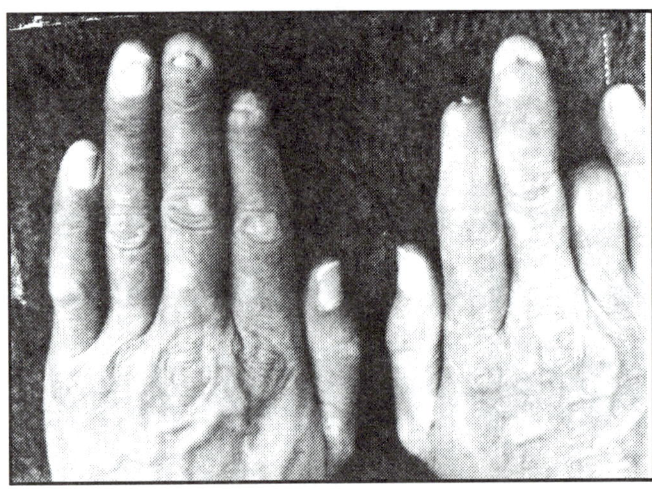

Fig. 19. Irregular finger length caused by resorption of the distal bony tufts. Note the absence of lesions on the Raynaud's patient's thumbs.

Because Raynaud's phenomenon can precede the other manifestations of limited cutaneous SSc by many years, it may be a valuable diagnostic clue. Raynaud's patients with abnormal or positive ANA, ESR, and/or nail-fold capillaroscopy test results are more prone to develop a rheumatic disease, especially SSc.[77,78] *(See also Appendix B.)*

Esophageal Hypomotility ("E" of the CREST Syndrome)

The esophagus is particularly susceptible to damage from SSc. The smooth muscles in the esophageal wall become scarred and fibrotic, which decreases peristalsis. In addition, patients commonly suffer esophageal hypomotility and gastroesophageal reflux, both of which can cause heartburn and solid food dysphagia.[78]

Sclerodactyly ("S" of the CREST Syndrome)

As the fatty tissues of the fingers and toes are replaced by abnormal amounts of collagen in SSc, the skin becomes indurated and tight; this condition is sclerodactyly (or acrosclerosis). As fibrosis tightens the skin overlying a finger or toe joint, patients develop flexion contractures. *(See Fig. 20.)* Tiny, painful ulcers may appear on the points of the elbows and the fingertips.

Other skin tissues become hard and shiny. Because the skin and/or epithelium are bound to underlying structures, patients have a characteristic drawn or hidebound appearance. The forehead is smooth and does not wrinkle; the subcutaneous tissues of the face shrink, and patients are left with the "classic expressionless face":[78] a pinched nose, puckered perioral skin, protruding teeth, and a fixed stare or grimace. Hyper- or hypopigmentation may occur. Ultimately, in the atrophic phase, the skin softens because of reduced subcutaneous fibrosis and thins because of reduced numbers of cutaneous capillary loops and resulting loss of subcutaneous tissue.[77]

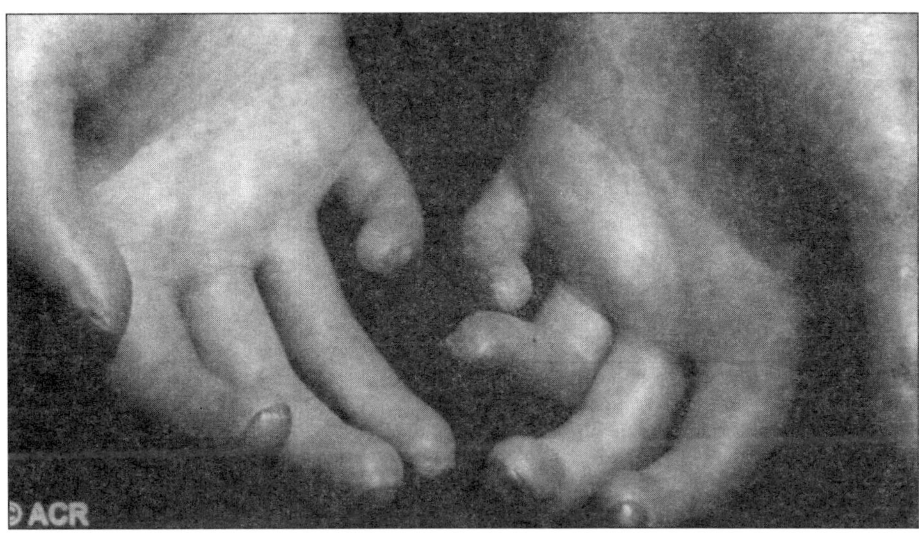

Fig. 20. Sclerodactyly has produced tightened, indurated skin and flexion contractures. Terminal digit resorption has shortened the second and third fingers.

Reprinted from the Clinical Slide Collection on the Rheumatic Diseases, *copyright 1991, 1995. Used by permission of the American College of Rheumatology.*

Telangiectasias ("T" of the CREST Syndrome)

Several years after onset of limited cutaneous SSc, patients often develop small, macular, punctate telangiectasias on their fingers, lips, tongue, oral mucous membranes, and/or face. *(See color plate A, page 49.)* However, because telangiectasias also appear in the late stages of diffuse cutaneous SSc, they are not, in themselves, indicative of limited cutaneous SSc.[83,86]

Oral Manifestations

Oral signs of SSc include restricted mouth opening and perioral wrinkles. (*See color plate A, page 49.*) Early mild edema of the tongue, soft palate, and larynx is followed by induration and atrophy of mucosal tissues. When the tongue becomes indurated and painful, patients often find it difficult to speak, chew, and/or swallow. Patients may also develop stiffness of the TMJ.[87] Since restricted mouth opening can result in inadequate home dental care, dental clinicians should instruct patients in perioral muscle exercises.[88]

Clinical Features of Diffuse Cutaneous SSc

As well as CREST syndrome, patients with diffuse cutaneous SSc have signs and symptoms indicating involvement of other organ systems. Careful monitoring of these systems can facilitate early recognition and treatment of SSc manifestations, which are discussed below.

Pulmonary Manifestations

Pulmonary disease is the primary cause of death for SSc patients.[77] Patients may report dyspnea on exertion, a nonproductive cough, and fatigue. Clinical examination may detect inspiratory crackles, particularly at the bases of the lungs. A high-resolution CAT scan may detect pulmonary alveolitis, an early inflammatory state which sometimes precedes the irreversible interstitial pulmonary fibrosis seen on radiographs. (*See Fig. 21.*) Weakening of diaphragm muscle fibers also interferes with respiration, causing pneumonitis or pulmonary insufficiency, which can lead to congestive heart failure. Patients with diffuse cutaneous SSc seldom have pulmonary arterial hypertension, which more often affects patients with limited cutaneous SSc.[77,78]

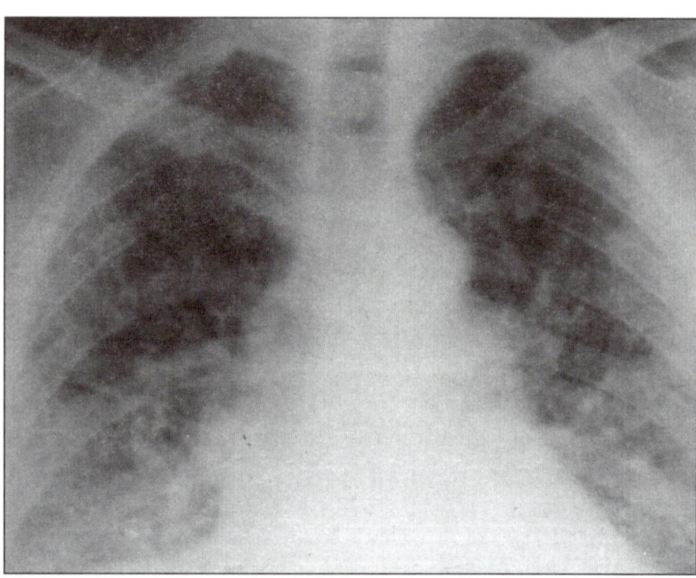

Fig. 21. Interstitial pulmonary fibrosis is a common manifestation of SSc and occurs in other rheumatic diseases; here, it produces "honeycomb" changes in the lower lung fields.

Reprinted from the Clinical Slide Collection on the Rheumatic Diseases, *copyright 1991, 1995. Used by permission of the American College of Rheumatology.*

Renal Manifestations

Renal crisis, involving malignant arterial hypertension, hyperreninemia, and renal failure, occurs in about 25% of patients with diffuse cutaneous SSc, often during the progressive skin-thickening phase within 4 years of onset of SSc.[83] Patients are at greatest risk for rapid deterioration if, within 3 days of renal crisis onset, their blood pressure is not effectively controlled and if, when treatment is started, they have creatinine levels >3 mg/dL.[89] Use of angiotensin-converting enzyme (ACE) inhibitors for rapid control of blood pressure has reduced the formerly high mortality rate among SSc patients in renal crisis.

GI Tract Manifestations

GI tract involvement can diminish the body's ability to digest and absorb nutrients and to eliminate wastes; patients may have cramping, bloating, diarrhea, or anorexia. Many patients report a dysphagic reaction to both solid foods and liquids. (*See also Esophageal Hypomotility in this chapter.*) In the small intestine, discontinuous smooth muscle function and dysmotility, which can cause bacterial overgrowth, may result in fat malabsorption.[77]

Cardiac Manifestations

Possible cardiac disorders include conduction disturbances, arrhythmias, and heart failure. Patients may report fatigue, chest pain, palpitations, and/or dyspnea.[77,78] In rare cases, SSc causes mitral stenosis or fibrinous pericarditis, leaving patients at risk for endocarditis. (*For patients requiring dental or other invasive procedures, see Endocarditis Prophylaxis, Chapter 6.*)

Secondary Conditions

Patients with SSc may be at increased risk for: (1) RA, SLE, and Sjögren's syndrome; and (2) cancer, with tumor sites corresponding to the sites commonly affected by fibrosis (e.g., lungs and skin).[90]

Treatment

Table 8 shows some of the drugs and therapeutic techniques currently used to treat manifestations of SSc. (*See Chapter 7 for discussions of other therapeutic techniques, including those used during dental care.*) Many agents have been employed to slow the progress of fibrosis in SSc. Unfortunately, only D-penicillamine has demonstrated efficacy, and even this drug is known to benefit only skin problems.[77]

Clinicians should instruct patients to take the following precautions:

1. Avoid exposure to cold by covering their hands and feet adequately before going outdoors
2. Avoid exposure to tobacco smoke, stressful situations, and any other potential causes of vasoconstriction

Table 8. Therapy for SSc

For potential adverse side effects of drugs, see appropriate algorithms in Chapter 6.

If a patient has:	Consider use of:
Arteriolar spasms and microcirculatory problems	• Vasodilator—to alleviate spasms of Raynaud's phenomenon: —Alpha-adrenergic receptor antagonist (e.g., prazosin)* —Calcium channel blocker (e.g., nifedipine)*[77,78] • Biofeedback—to retrain the finger capillaries to dilate, not constrict, in response to cold • Physical activity, especially light exercise and continuing movement of the fingers and joints—to inhibit development of stiffness and contracture
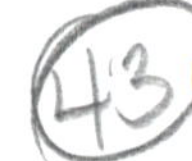 Cutaneous fibrosis	• D-penicillamine—to interfere with collagen metabolism • Methotrexate (MTX)—still experimental, though promising 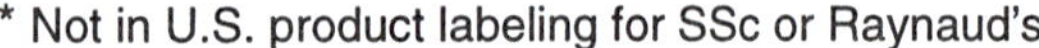
GI tract manifestations	• Metoclopramide—to stimulate peristalsis • H_2-receptor antagonist (e.g. cimetidine) or the gastric acid pump inhibitor omeprazole—to treat severe gastroesophageal reflux and dyspepsia • Antibiotic (e.g., tetracycline)—to treat bacterial overgrowth within the small intestine • Supplemental nutrition—to treat weight loss and anorexia
Hypomobility	• Physical therapy—to maintain joint mobility and prevent worsening of flexion contractures[77]
Interstitial pulmonary fibrosis	• Oral cyclophosphamide during early inflammatory stages—to improve symptoms and vital capacity[91] *(See also Immunosuppressants, Chapter 6.)*
Pruritus	• Combined Type I and II histamine blocker; topical moisturizer—to relieve itching[77]
Pulmonary hypertension	• Calcium channel blocker (e.g., nifedipine) and supplemental oxygen—to improve symptoms (but not necessarily affect disease course)[92]
Renal crisis	• ACE inhibitor (e.g., captopril)*—to control blood pressure rapidly and to reverse hyperreninemia[77,78,83]

* Not in U.S. product labeling for SSc or Raynaud's

3. Reduce gastroesophageal reflux, by:
   a. Taking oral liquid-form drugs, or, as an alternative, crushing tablets and swallowing them with water
   b. Eating several small meals per day
   c. Taking antacids between meals
   d. Eating their evening meals an hour or more before bedtime
   e. Abstaining from caffeine (e.g., coffee, tea, chocolate)
   f. Sleeping on two pillows or elevating the heads of beds on wooden blocks
4. Follow up regularly with a health care provider for general assessment of disease progression, including blood pressure monitoring and pulmonary function testing.

Clinicians and patients can contact agencies listed in Appendix A to obtain further information.

Prognosis

The prognosis for SSc depends upon the extent and distribution of organ involvement, and upon the rapidity of the disease's progression.[77] When diffuse cutaneous SSc involves the lungs, heart, and/or kidneys, death can occur early in the course of the disease. When limited cutaneous SSc includes less dramatic organ involvement, prognosis is better. The overall 10-year survival rate, after diagnosis, is approximately 65%.[83]

Chapter Summary

1. Systemic sclerosis (SSc), sometimes called "scleroderma," is characterized by fibrosis and microvascular injury.
2. In limited cutaneous SSc, skin thickening is confined to the face, neck and extremities, Raynaud's is present for years to decades, and systemic manifestations occur late in the disease course.
3. In diffuse cutaneous SSc, skin thickening occurs on the trunk as well as the face, neck, and extremities, and organ system involvement occurs early in the disease course.
4. Females are three to eight times more susceptible than men to idiopathic SSc.
5. Limited cutaneous SSc is also known as the CREST syndrome, which includes: (1) calcinosis; (2) Raynaud's phenomenon; (3) esophageal hypomotility; (4) sclerodactyly; and (5) telangiectasia.
6. A significant percentage of patients with limited cutaneous SSc ultimately develops pulmonary arterial hypertension, which has a poor prognosis.
7. Raynaud's phenomenon, the initial complaint in about 70% of SSc patients, is a circulatory system disorder affecting the fingers and, occasionally, the toes.
8. Systemic manifestations of diffuse cutaneous SSc can include: (1) pulmonary interstitial fibrosis; (2) renal crisis; (3) GI tract problems (e.g., cramping; diarrhea; anorexia); and (4) cardiac disorders (e.g., arrhythmias; heart failure).
9. D-penicillamine has been shown to slow the progress of skin fibrosis in SSc patients.
10. Clinicians should caution patients with SSc to: (1) avoid exposure to cold and vasoconstrictors; (2) take precautions to reduce gastroesophageal reflux; and (3) have a health care provider monitor the disease course regularly.

Progress Test E

1. Two main subgroups of systemic sclerosis (SSc) are ______________ cutaneous SSc and ___________ cutaneous SSc.

2. Incidence of SSc peaks in persons from about _____ to _____ years old.

3. The major criterion used as a diagnostic guide for SSc is ________________ scleroderma.

4. Tendon friction rubs are generally found in patients with ___________ cutaneous SSc.

5. ________________, in which calcium salts are deposited in the skin, usually appears long after other SSc signs and symptoms have emerged.

6. The fingers of patients with Raynaud's phenomenon turn pale when _________________ ___________ causes small arteries to constrict.

7. When smooth muscles in the esophageal wall become scarred and fibrotic, ____________________ is decreased.

8. Perioral ____________ ________________ can benefit SSc patients with restricted mouth opening.

9. ________ _________________ must be effectively controlled within 3 days of onset of renal crisis.

10. To reduce gastroesophageal reflux, patients should eat their evening meals ____ ________ ____ ________ before bedtime.

Chapter 6 Pharmacotherapies

Patients with rheumatic disorders are given pharmacotherapy to reduce inflammation, relieve pain, combat infections, alleviate insomnia, and treat other manifestations. The current approach is to make patients as comfortable as possible, quickly, using whichever drugs work best with acceptable side effects. Some patients (e.g., those with Raynaud's phenomenon) may need to crush tablets and dissolve them in water in order to swallow them.

Since most patients with rheumatic disorders require pharmacotherapy indefinitely, they must be closely and regularly monitored for complications.

This chapter summarizes the adverse side effects which can be produced by drugs used to treat the six rheumatic diseases/syndromes discussed in this course. For more complete data on drug use and side effects, clinicians can consult appropriate journals and references (e.g., *Facts and Comparisons,* the *USP Dispensing Information/USP DI*, etc.). To avoid serious drug interactions, all clinicians should determine which drugs (prescription and over-the-counter) each patient is already taking, before prescribing or using others during treatment. Since most patients with rheumatic disorders require pharmacotherapy indefinitely, they must be closely and regularly monitored for complications.

Disease-Modifying Antirheumatic Drugs

Disease-modifying antirheumatic drugs (DMARDs) are used to treat RA which remains active despite treatment with NSAIDs. (*See also RA Treatment: Pharmacotherapy, Chapter 1.*) Certain DMARDs also benefit patients with SLE and SSc, as discussed below.

Algorithm 11 shows potential adverse side effects of DMARDs and the ACR's recommendations on how to monitor patients taking these drugs. Several DMARDs can produce fetal abnormalities, and, when taking a DMARD contraindicated for pregnant patients, women of childbearing age should use effective contraception.[2, 93]

Immunosuppressants

Azathioprine (AZA): This drug is used to treat RA when patients cannot tolerate other DMARDs. It is also used to reduce immune system activity in patients with SLE, although it is not included in U.S. product labeling for that disease. Algorithm 11 shows some side effects of AZA.

AZA can suppress bone marrow activity at dosages of 1 to 2 mg per kg per day.

AZA can suppress bone marrow activity (myelosuppression) at dosages of 1 to 2 mg per kg per day.[93] To decrease the incidence or severity of myelosuppression and its complications (bleeding, severe anemia, sepsis), the ACR recommends that patients taking AZA have a CBC and platelet count every 1 to 2 weeks until the dosage is stabilized, and every 1 to 3 months thereafter. Patients with renal insufficiency who take AZA are at higher risk for myelosuppression; this risk is also increased for patients who take allopurinol or ACE inhibitors and AZA concurrently. The ACR recommends the following measures to prevent myelosuppression:

1. Decreasing the AZA dosage for patients with renal insufficiency
2. Reducing the AZA dosage to one fourth the usual dosage when allopurinol is used concurrently
3. Avoiding the use of ACE inhibitors for patients receiving AZA.[2,93]

AZA is contraindicated for pregnant patients because of risks of intrauterine growth retardation and prematurity and, in neonates, transient immunosuppression.[2,93]

Cyclophosphamide: This immunosuppressant <u>may</u> be prescribed for refractory RA or for severe extraarticular manifestations of rheumatic diseases, including: (1) glomerulonephritis caused by SLE (*see Table 5*); and (2) interstitial pulmonary fibrosis caused by SSc (*see Table 8*).

Cyclophosphamide (e.g., Cytoxan®), which, with long-term use or high doses, can produce acute myopericarditis or hemorrhagic cystitis, is not included in U.S. product labeling for RA, SLE, or SSc; if use of the drug is deemed necessary, it should be administered only by rheumatologists experienced in monitoring it.[93]

D-Penicillamine

D-penicillamine was first isolated as a component of penicillin; today, it is produced synthetically. D-penicillamine is most often used for RA patients with extraarticular manifestations. It may also help to slow skin fibrosis and hardening in patients with SSc. However, the drug can, in rare cases, produce several adverse side effects. (*See Algorithm 11.*) The ACR recommends a CBC and a urinalysis for protein every 2

Algorithm 11. Using Six Types of DMARDs		
When prescribing:	**Remember these adverse side effects:**	**And monitor for:**
Azathioprine (AZA): Imuran®	• **Common:** Gastrointestinal intolerance; myelosuppression • **Infrequent:** hepatotoxicity • **Rare:** pancreatitis	• Bone marrow activity • Hepatic function
D-penicillamine: Cuprimine® Depen®	• **Common:** distorted sense of taste; rash; stomatitis • **Rare:** Goodpasture's syndrome; myasthenia gravis; polymyositis; proteinuria; renal failure; thrombocytopenia	• Bone marrow activity • Edema • Hematuria • Proteinuria • Rash
Gold compounds: • I.M. aurothiomalate: Myochrysine® • I.M. aurothioglucose: Solganol® • Oral auranofin: Ridaura®	• **Common:** oral ulcers; rash • **Infrequent:** pruritus without rash • **Rare:** aplastic anemia; interstitial pneumonitis; membranous glomerulonephritis; thrombocytopenia • (**With oral auranofin:** diarrhea)	• Bone marrow activity • Edema • Hematuria • Oral ulcers • Proteinuria • Rash
Hydroxychloroquine (HCQ): Plaquenil®	• **Rare:** abnormal skin pigmentation; blurred vision; gastrointestinal intolerance; myopathy; peripheral neuropathy; retinal damage	• Ocular changes (eye exams every 6 to 12 months)
Methotrexate (MTX): Folex® Rheumatrex®	• **Common:** gastrointestinal disturbances; mild alopecia; mucositis • **Rare:** cirrhosis; hepatic fibrosis; hypersensitivity pneumonitis; myelosuppression	• Bone marrow activity • Dyspnea • Lymph node swelling • Nausea/vomiting
Sulfasalazine (SSZ): Azulfidine®	• **Common:** abdominal pain; anorexia; dyspepsia; headache; mood alteration; nausea/vomiting; photosensitivity; rash • **Infrequent:** leukopenia • **Rare:** agranulocytosis; aplastic or hemolytic anemia; thrombocytopenia; myelosuppression; hepatitis	• Bone marrow activity • Photosensitivity • Rash

weeks until the dosage is stable, then every 1 to 3 months. A slow increase in the D-penicillamine dosage—by 125 to 250 mg increments every 3 months up to 750 mg per day—seems to decrease the incidence of thrombocytopenia.[2,93]

D-penicillamine is highly reactive with certain drugs.

D-penicillamine is highly reactive with certain drugs (e.g., phenylbutazone, cytotoxic drugs, and gold compounds). At least 2 hours should elapse between its administration and that of any other drug or vitamins. D-penicillamine is contraindicated for patients with LE, a previous penicillamine-induced hematologic disease, or a history of renal insufficiency. Because it can produce fetal connective tissue abnormalities, it is also contraindicated for pregnant patients and those considering pregnancy.

Gold Compounds

Chrysotherapy, used for RA and psoriatic arthritis, can be administered orally or by intramuscular (I.M.) injection. Algorithm 11 shows adverse side effects of chrysotherapy. Thrombocytopenia and aplastic anemia may occur suddenly. Membranous glomerulonephritis is usually heralded by hematuria or proteinuria.[2,93]

The ACR recommends that patients receiving I.M. gold have a CBC, platelet count, and urinalysis every 1 to 2 weeks for the first 20 weeks, then at the time of subsequent (or alternate) injections. Patients taking gold orally should have these laboratory tests every 4 to 12 weeks. The ACR also recommends that patients with qualitative proteinuria undergo a 24-hour urinalysis and, if protein excretion is >500 mg/24 hours, physicians should consider stopping chrysotherapy.[2,93]

Hydroxychloroquine

For reasons yet unknown, the antimalarial agent hydroxychloroquine (HCQ) modulates the symptoms of SLE and RA, and, compared with other DMARDs, is the least costly to monitor and the least toxic; however, breastfeeding is contraindicated. HCQ is sometimes used in combination with methotrexate, sulfasalazine, glucocorticoids, and/or aspirin; the dosage of all the drugs can often be reduced when they are combined.

> Patients taking HCQ should report any difficulty seeing entire faces or printed words, decreased night vision, loss of peripheral vision, or intolerance to glare.

Algorithm 11 shows rare HCQ adverse side effects. Retinal complications most often occur when patients >70 years take a cumulative HCQ dosage of >800 gm; increased risk of these complications, particularly for patients with abnormal hepatic or renal function, may also be associated with a daily HCQ dosage of >6.0 to 6.5 mg per kg. Clinicians should caution patients taking HCQ to report any difficulty seeing entire faces or printed words, decreased night vision, loss of peripheral vision, or intolerance to glare. Patients with these symptoms should stop taking HCQ, be evaluated by an ophthalmologist, and be given an Amsler test (HCQ-produced retinal damage begins in the central 10° of the visual field, and Amsler's charts are used to detect central visual field defects). The ACR recommends that ophthalmologic evaluations be performed every 6 to 12 months for most patients, but more frequently for those who have taken HCQ >10 years or have abnormal renal function.[2,93]

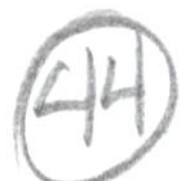

Methotrexate

For patients with severe RA, many physicians select methotrexate (MTX), an antimetabolite, as the initial DMARD. Patients with SSc may also benefit from MTX with slowing of skin fibrosis. Although generally well tolerated, MTX can produce hepatic fibrosis and cirrhosis *(see Algorithm 11)*, especially in patients who drink alcoholic beverages. Patients taking MTX must be reminded frequently to avoid even small amounts of beer, wine, or hard liquor. All patients should report occurrences of dark urine or jaundice. The ACR recommends liver biopsies only as a pretreatment precaution for patients with suspected liver disease, and for patients with hepatic function abnormalities which persist during treatment with, or following discontinuation of, MTX.[2,93]

> Because MTX has antimetabolic effects, women who are, or may become, pregnant must avoid it.

The ACR recommends that patients taking MTX have a CBC, platelet count, and tests for levels of serum aspartate aminotransferase (AST), albumin, and creatinine every 4 to 8 weeks. Patients at particular risk for MTX-produced myelosuppression include those with renal insufficiency or folate deficiency and those taking antifolate agents (e.g., trimethoprim). In addition, because MTX has antimetabolic effects, women who are, or may become, pregnant must avoid it. The drug can cause spontaneous abortions, as well as fetal abnormalities (e.g., cleft palate and hydrocephalus).[2,93]

Long-term MTX therapy can rarely produce hypersensitivity pneumonitis. The ACR recommends that, within 1 year of initiating MTX, a patient have an x-ray to determine if significant lung disease is present; if it is, MTX therapy should be reconsidered. Less serious side effects of MTX (e.g., mucositis, alopecia, and gastrointestinal disturbances) may be caused by folate depletion; therefore, the ACR recommends that all patients taking MTX be given folic acid (1 mg per day or 7 mg once a week). Because a few case reports suggest a possible association between MTX and lymphoma, the ACR recommends that primary care physicians routinely examine lymph nodes of patients taking MTX.[2,93]

Sulfasalazine

Sulfasalazine (SSZ), used specifically to treat RA, is a relatively safe and effective alternative to other DMARDs. The mechanism by which this drug exerts its beneficial effect is not clear. Even though SSZ's aspirin component passes through the GI tract without being absorbed, it can irritate GI tract tissue; therefore, many patients take enteric-coated SSZ tablets. Patients with glucose 6-phosphate dehydrogenase (G6PD) deficiency and/or blood diseases are at risk for the rare hematologic side effects of SSZ. *(See Algorithm 11.)* Stevens-Johnson syndrome, a severe hypersensitivity reaction involving skin and mucous membranes, may develop in patients allergic to sulfa drugs; therefore, any history of allergy to Septra®, Bactrim®, or related drugs contraindicates SSZ use.

The ACR recommends that CBCs be done every 2 to 4 weeks for the first 3 months of SSZ therapy, and every 3 months thereafter. The ACR also suggests establishing a baseline AST serum level for patients with known or suspected hepatic disease; other experts advise regular screening of hepatic function because some patients taking SSZ have developed hepatitis. Because of the risk of fetal kernicterus, SSZ is contraindicated in late-term pregnancy.[2,93]

Glucocorticoids

Glucocorticoids (systemic corticosteroids) have excellent anti-inflammatory effects, and often relieve symptoms of RA and many systemic manifestations of SLE. However, they do not modify the course of a rheumatic disease,[23] and their long-term use is fraught with toxicity. (*See Pharmacotherapy, Chapter 1; Table 5, Chapter 3.*)

Algorithm 12 shows many of the adverse side effects which glucocorticoids can produce. Physicians prescribing glucocorticoids should advise patients to reduce their cholesterol intake and, if they smoke, to quit, so as to minimize the tendency for accelerated atherogenesis. The ACR recommends that decisions to use these drugs take into account predisposing factors for adverse side effects, including:

1. Established hypertension or diabetes (or a family history of diabetes)
2. Preexisting glaucoma or cataracts
3. A history of osteoporotic fracture, documented low bone mineral density, or premature menopause.[2]

Algorithm 12. Using Glucocorticoids

When prescribing:	Remember these adverse side effects:	And monitor for:
• **Methylprednisolone:** Depo-Predate® Medrol® • **Prednisolone:** Predate® Predcor® • **Prednisone:** Deltasone® Orasone®	• Atherosclerosis • Avascular necrosis of bone • Cataract formation • Diabetes • Glaucoma • Hypertension • Impaired wound healing • Increased susceptibility to infection • Osteoporosis	• Abnormal glucose levels • Edema • Elevated blood pressure • Excessive thirst • New bone or joint pain • Polyuria • Visual changes

Glucocorticoids must be administered cautiously: the oral dosage is gradually increased until the patient improves, then is tapered off and eventually discontinued if possible. Generally, these drugs are used only for short periods; when patients require oral glucocorticoids over longer periods, alternate-day dosing regimens are often used to minimize side

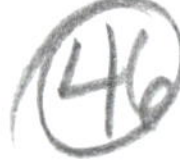

effects. Patients receiving long-term glucocorticoid therapy should wear a medical alert bracelet. All patients taking these drugs should be under close medical supervision; Algorithm 12 shows the ACR's recommendations on how to monitor such patients.[2]

At times, systemic steroids may be avoided through the use of topical steroids. For example, when the rheumatic disease is under control but one or two joints remain inflamed and painful, an injection of glucocorticoid into the affected intraarticular space often reduces the inflammation and relieves the pain. The effect can last from a few weeks to several months, and, since the drug remains within the joint, systemic side effects are minimal.

Nonsteroidal Anti-Inflammatory Drugs

Nonsteroidal anti-inflammatory drugs (NSAIDs) reduce pain, swelling, and fever, but do not prevent joint destruction or alter the courses of rheumatic diseases. NSAIDs comprise two groups: those containing salicylates (aspirin) and those without it.

A synergistic reaction can occur when two or more NSAIDs are combined.

Algorithm 13 shows adverse side effects of NSAIDs, although all but dyspepsia are either infrequent or rare. Because a synergistic (or additive) reaction—resulting in greater toxicity—can occur when two or more NSAIDs are combined, patients should be advised to avoid such combinations. The ACR recommends that, before deciding to prescribe NSAIDs, physicians consider whether patients are at risk for:

1. Gastrointestinal complications, which can affect patients already using glucocorticoids, those with cardiovascular disease or a history of peptic ulcers, and the elderly
2. Renal complications, which can affect patients with renal disease, cirrhosis, or congestive heart failure, and the elderly (especially those already taking diuretics).

Algorithm 13. Using NSAIDs

When prescribing:	Remember these adverse side effects:	And monitor for:
• Aspirin: Ecotrin®; Bayer®; Anacin®; Excedrin® • Ibuprofen: Motrin®; Advil® • Indomethacin: Indocin® • Naproxen: Aleve®; Naprosyn® • Piroxicam: Feldene® • Sulindac: Clinoril®	• **Common**: dyspepsia • **Infrequent:** gastrointestinal bleeding or ulceration; myelosuppression; prolonged bleeding time; proteinuria • **Rare:** confusion; depression; headache; hepatotoxicity; rash; renal insufficiency	• Abdominal pain • Black/dark stool • Dyspepsia • Easy bruising • Edema • Nausea/vomiting

Aspirin generally has to be taken more frequently than other NSAIDs, but is well tolerated by most patients. Further, since aspirin costs less than other NSAIDs, it is particularly favored by patients without prescription drug insurance coverage. Using enteric-coated aspirin (Ecotrin®) and taking aspirin with food, antacids, and ≥8 ounces of water are often recommended to protect patients from gastric mucosal irritation. However, antacids and histamine H_2-receptor antagonists can mask heartburn (an initial ulcer symptom), and developing ulcers in such patients may go unrecognized because the symptom is not reported. Patients with a documented history of peptic ulcers, gastrointestinal bleeding, or cardiovascular disease should take misoprostol (Cytotec®), a gastric mucosa protectant, if they must use an NSAID.[2,93]

Algorithm 13 shows the ACR's recommendations on how to monitor patients taking NSAIDs; clinicians should also do a yearly CBC. Patients concurrently taking diuretics or ACE inhibitors should undergo weekly serum creatinine tests for at least 3 weeks. Hepatic function should be monitored as well, especially in patients with intrinsic hepatic disease.[2,93]

Pregnant patients should try to avoid NSAIDs, particularly in the third trimester; these drugs cross the placenta and may produce fetal complications (e.g., premature arterial duct closure, which can cause pulmonary hypertension).[2,93]

Other Systemic Drugs

Algorithm 14 shows some potential side effects of other systemic drugs suggested as treatments for the six rheumatic diseases/syndromes discussed in this coursebook. As mentioned previously, clinicians are advised to consult pharmaceutical references (e.g., *Facts and Comparisons,* the *USP Dispensing Information/ USP DI*, etc.).

Endocarditis Prophylaxis

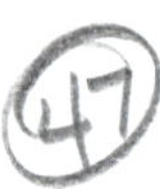

Before scheduling oral, esophageal, respiratory tract, GI tract, or genitourinary tract procedures, clinicians should determine if patients with cardiac defects need prophylactic antibiotics to prevent bacterial endocarditis. Current information on how to make this decision can be found in:

1. Dajani AS, Taubert KA, Wilson W, et al. Prevention of bacterial endocarditis: recommendations by the American Heart Association. *JAMA.* June 11, 1997;277(22):1794-1801.
2. Dajani AS, Taubert KA, Wilson W, et al. Prevention of bacterial endocarditis: recommendations by the American Heart Association. *JADA.* August 1997;128:1142-1151.

Algorithm 14. Other Systemic Drugs			
When prescribing:	**Such as:***	**For:**	**Remember these side effects:**
ACE inhibitor	Captopril: Capoten®	Hypertension *(esp. in SSc—see renal crisis, Table 8)*	• Proteinuria can occur with doses of >150 mg/day • Hypotension; rash; fever; arthralgia
Analgesic	Acetaminophen: Tylenol®	Pain *(esp. in FMS—see Algorithm 6)*	• Rare: agranulocytosis; dermatitis; anemia; hepatitis; renal failure; thrombocytopenia
Alpha-adrenergic receptor antagonist	Prazosin: Minipress®	Raynaud's *(esp. in SSc—see arteriolar spasms, Table 8)*	• Hypotensive reaction, including dizziness (start prazosin therapy at lowest possible dose to lessen chances of this reaction) • Lower limb swelling; heart palpitations; urinary incontinence
Anabolic steroid	Danazol: Danocrine®	Angioedema prophylaxis *(esp. in SLE—see thrombocytopenia, Table 5)*	• Disruption and/or irregularity of menstrual period
Benzodiazepine sedative-hypnotic	Alprazolam: Xanax® Zolpidem: Ambien®	Anxiety *(esp. in FMS—see Algorithm 6)*	• Confusion; depression (alprazolam) • Ataxia; confusion; depression (zolpidem)
Calcium channel blocker	Nifedipine: Procardia®	Hypertension *(esp. in SLE—see renal m.; in SSc—see Table 8);* and for Raynaud's *(esp. in SSc—see Table 8)*	• Dizziness; dyspnea; headache; irregular heartbeat; hypotension; extremity swelling
Dermatitis modifier	Dapsone: Avlosulfon®	Discoid rash *(esp. in SLE—see cutaneous manifestations, Table 5)*	• Agranulocytosis; aplastic anemia; cyanosis; rash
Nontricyclic antidepressant	Fluoxetine: Prozac®	Fatigue; depression *(esp. in FMS—see Algorithm 6)*	• Arthralgia; dyspnea; fever; myalgia; rash
Gastric acid pump inhibitor	Omeprazole	Reflux; dyspepsia *(esp. in SSc—see GI tract, Table 8)*	• Rare: anemia; leukocytosis; oral ulcers; bloody or cloudy urine
Histamine H_2-receptor antagonist	Cimetidine: Tagamet®	Reflux; dyspepsia *(esp. in SSc—see GI tract, Table 8)*	• Hypotension (caused by rapid I.V. administration) • Rare: arrhythmia; hepatitis
Peristaltic stimulant	Metoclopramide: Propulsid®	GI dysmotility *(esp. in SSc—see GI tract, Table 8)*	• Rare: agranulocytosis; hypotension; irregular heartbeat; uncontrolled limb movements
Phenothiazine antipsychotic	Perphenazine: Trilafon®	Pain amplification *(esp. in FMS—see Algorithm 6)*	• Blurred vision; hypotension; muscle spasms; restlessness; uncontrolled limb movements
Skeletal muscle relaxant	Cyclobenzaprine: Flexeril®	Muscle spasm *(esp. in FMS—see Algorithm 6)*	• Drowsiness • Rare: anaphylaxis; confusion; depression; hive-like facial swelling on face; rash
Cytokine inhibitor	Thalidomide: Synovir™	Oral discoid lesions *(esp. in SLE—see Table 5)*	• Neuropathy • Rare: bone marrow suppression
Tricyclic antidepressants	Amitriptyline: Elavil® Doxepin: Sinequan®	Sleep disorders; pain amplification *(esp. in CFS—see CFS Treatment; and FMS—see Algorithm 6)*	• Blurred vision; confusion; constipation; difficult urination; irregular heartbeat; hypotension; nervousness; tremors

* Representative generic and brand names are given.

Chapter Summary

1. To avoid serious drug interactions, all clinicians should determine which prescription and over-the counter drugs each patient is already taking before prescribing or using others during treatment.

2. Since most patients with rheumatic disorders require pharmacotherapy indefinitely, they must be closely and regularly monitored for adverse side effects.

3. Disease-modifying antirheumatic drugs (DMARDs) are used to treat RA which remains active despite treatment with NSAIDs; certain DMARDs also benefit patients with SLE and SSc.

4. Many DMARDs can produce fetal abnormalities, so women should avoid pregnancy when taking these drugs.

5. Azathioprine (AZA) may be used to treat RA when patients cannot tolerate other DMARDs, but it often causes myelosuppression.

6. The DMARD D-penicillamine, used to treat patients with RA and SSc, is highly reactive with other drugs, including gold compounds.

7. Rare side effects of gold compounds, used to treat RA, include thrombocytopenia and aplastic anemia, which may occur suddenly.

8. Hydroxychloroquine (HCQ) relieves the symptoms of SLE and RA; however, certain patients may be at risk for retinal complications.

9. Methotrexate (MTX) is often selected as the initial DMARD for patients with severe RA; patients taking this drug must avoid alcoholic beverages.

10. Sulfasalazine (SSZ), used to treat RA, is a relatively safe and effective alternative to other DMARDs.

11. Glucocorticoids, which often relieve RA symptoms and certain SLE systemic manifestations, must be administered cautiously because the adverse side effects they produce can manifest as serious complications.

12. Nonsteroidal anti-inflammatory drugs (NSAIDs) reduce pain, swelling, and fever, but do not prevent joint destruction.

Progress Test F

1. Patients who take AZA concurrently with allopurinol or ACE inhibitors have increased risk for ______________________.

2. With long-term use or high doses, ______________________ can produce acute myopericarditis or hemorrhagic cystitis.

3. Patients taking gold compounds by intramuscular injection should have a CBC, platelet count, and urinalysis every 1 to 2 weeks for the first _____ __________.

4. Patients taking HCQ and experiencing vision difficulties should stop taking the drug, be evaluated by an ophthalmologist, and be given an __________ test.

5. Drinking alcoholic beverages is prohibited for patients taking ______ because this drug can produce hepatic fibrosis and cirrhosis.

6. SSZ is contraindicated in late-term pregnancy because of the risk of ________ __________________.

7. To minimize vascular problems, patients taking glucocorticoids should reduce their ________________ intake and refrain from __________.

8. Some NSAIDs contain _________________ (____________); others do not.

9. Patients with a history of peptic ulcers, gastrointestinal bleeding, or cardiovascular disease should take ________________ concurrently with NSAIDs.

10. ______________ ____________________ used to treat CFS and FMS can produce blurred vision, irregular heartbeat, hypotension, and tremors.

Chapter 7 Nondrug Therapies

The six rheumatic disorders discussed in this coursebook cause pain, interfere with patients' abilities to work, change their appearances, and bar them from many leisure activities. Afflicted patients find it difficult to lift, bend, twist, or climb. These physical problems greatly impair their overall well-being and ability to adhere to a regular schedule of personal care.

The long-term consequences for young people with rheumatic disorders are often closely tied to their level of education.

Effects of rheumatic disorders on patients' abilities to perform routine tasks, in turn, have an impact on their standard of living. Illnesses which begin in childhood (e.g., JRA) may necessitate frequent school absences, interfering with educational progress. Carrying books, writing, and even getting to and from classes are also affected. Furthermore, the long-term consequences for young people with rheumatic disorders are often closely tied to their level of education. Jobs which require less schooling (e.g., manual labor, secretarial positions, and various service positions) may be out of the question for people suffering sequelae of RA, SLE, or SSc. Those who manage to achieve higher levels of education are most likely to qualify for occupations requiring perseverance and intellectual striving, qualities unaffected by rheumatic disorders; these occupations elevate patients' socioeconomic status. Patients who are disabled should be reminded that the Americans with Disabilities Act of 1990 protects them from discrimination by employers.

Reassuring Patients

Psychologic effects of rheumatic disorders can manifest as anger and depression, both of which may aggravate patients' physical symptoms. Many patients benefit from participation in local support groups (e.g., the Arthritis Foundation offers a 6-week "Arthritis Self-Help Course"; patients learn to participate more actively in their arthritis care). Patients can locate local support groups by checking local telephone directories or by calling any of the numbers in Appendix A.

Clinicians should assure patients that periods of exacerbation are seldom totally disabling. They can also boost patients' morale by showing them concern, encouraging them to discuss their frustrations, and helping them to alleviate their pain and discomfort.

Relieving Pain and Discomfort

The simplest way to relieve pain is to apply cold or heat to the affected area, preferably under the guidance of a physical therapist. Rest also helps to reduce pain, but patients should achieve an optimal balance between rest and exercise. (*See Exercising Appropriately.*) Algorithm 15 shows various nondrug techniques used to relieve, avoid, or minimize pain and discomfort.[84]

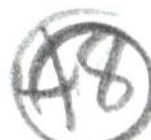

Algorithm 15. Nondrug Treatment of Pain and Discomfort		
If patient has:	**Suggest that patient:**	**Which:**
Pain caused by an acute inflammatory reaction	• Apply cold to the affected area, using a refrigerated moist pack or ice bag for no longer than 10 to 20 minutes Note: *Patients should not use a cold pack if they have sensitivity to cold; decreased sensation; decreased circulation; and/or cardiovascular problems.*	Acts on pain receptors as an analgesic, and counteracts muscle spasm
Pain which is chronic	• Apply heat to the affected area, using a heating pad or hot compress wrapped in towels for no longer than 10 to 30 minutes; the skin should be dry (no lotions/creams), and checked every 5 minutes for signs of burning • Take a warm bath or shower • Use diathermy (infrared lamp) • Use hot paraffin only under the supervision of a therapist Note: *Patients should not apply heat if they have sensitivity to heat; decreased sensation; and/or decreased circulation.*	Relieves discomfort, stiffness, inflammation, and spasms
Pain of any type	• Rest by lying quietly on a firm mattress with no more than one pillow, keeping the spine straight, or, if going to bed is not possible, relaxing in a chair for ≥15 minutes Note: *Lying on either side with knees bent helps some patients, but those with shoulder or hip involvement find this position uncomfortable.*	Relieves pain by preventing muscle spasm and joint stress
Pain of any type while doing unavoidable tasks	• Do unavoidable, painful tasks the easy way (e.g., slide objects rather than carry them) • Organize work so that materials are within reach, with the work counter at a comfortable height • Do most work as quickly as possible, while seated, with fingers relaxed and extended; several times a day, massage and rest the hands and fingers for a few minutes	Reduces pain

The suggestions in Algorithm 15 are to be followed only as temporary adjuncts to the pharmacotherapy and other treatment prescribed by patients' primary care physicians or rheumatologists.[84] Clinicians should encourage patients to take the prescribed doses of their drug regimens, even during periods of relative comfort. Many drugs work slowly, so benefits are apparent only after weeks or months of regular use. Similarly, the deterioration associated with noncompliance may not become noticeable for weeks.

Relieving Stress on Joints

Stress on joints can worsen pain and inflammation. Patients can avoid joint stress by:

1. Maintaining normal weight; obesity places stress on all weight-bearing joints
2. Maintaining proper posture (e.g., keeping upper back straight when sitting or standing; squatting when lifting objects); poor posture puts stress on the spine, neck, and shoulders
3. Using ergometric aids (e.g., sleeping on the side, not on the stomach or back; using a footstool to keep the knees higher than the hips when sitting; using a footstool to raise one foot slightly when standing for a long time; wearing shoes with thick rubber soles)
4. Taking occasional breaks, changing position frequently, and using helpful devices—when they must lift, twist, reach, and/or stand or sit in one place for long periods.

Clinicians should encourage patients to avoid, when possible, tasks that always cause pain (e.g., carrying heavy loads), require force, or necessitate repetitive or twisting movements.

Promoting Oral Health

Clinical Care

Because patients with rheumatic diseases often have dry and tender oral tissues, their teeth should be cleaned professionally every 3 to 4 months. Ultrasonic scalers can be used if the teeth and gums are not too sensitive, but coarse polish and acidic fluoride gel should be avoided. Fine polishing paste and neutral fluoride gel should be used on patients with delicate mucous membranes.

During dental care, patients with rheumatic disorders must be given frequent rest periods, so that they can close their mouths, change their sitting positions, and relax aching muscles. Scheduling extra time allows practitioners to offer optimal therapy and patients to suffer less discomfort and anxiety. Patients with TMJ and esophageal problems require further consideration.

TMJ problems: Lengthy dental procedures can stress the TMJ to the point of causing extreme pain. Nonemergency dental treatment should be postponed if patients are suffering acute pain in this joint. They may obtain relief from chronic TMJ pain by wearing a bite support appliance, which decompresses the joint and repositions the condyle-disk assembly. Applying moist heat to the sides of their face helps relieve occasional TMJ pain.

Esophageal problems: Patients suffering esophageal manifestations of a rheumatic disease (e.g., SSc patients) should not be put in supine positions for long periods while a dental drill sprays water on the back of their throats. The symptoms of esophageal hypomotility and gastroesophageal reflux worsen when a patient lies flat or bends over.

Home Care

At home, patients should brush with fluoride toothpaste and an extra-soft toothbrush, using a child-sized one if necessary. Patients who can floss should do so at least once a day. Water irrigators, used on the lowest power, are acceptable for patients with no cardiac complications, but only if their tender oral tissues will not suffer from the treatment. Patients who find it difficult to grasp, manipulate, or control a toothbrush or dental floss should be advised to try devices discussed in Chapter 8.

> Before purchasing mouth rinses, patients should check the labels for "active ingredients," particularly alcohol content.

Patients can benefit from use of chlorhexidine gluconate (Peridex®), a prescription antiseptic rinse, or over-the-counter fluoride mouth rinses. Before purchasing such products, patients should check the labels for "active ingredients"; the alcohol content of popular mouth rinses ranges from 7% to 21.6%; those with no alcohol content include Clear Choice® and Rembrandt®. Clinicians should advise patients to avoid all products containing alcohol and other ingredients which can dry or irritate mucosal tissues.

Preventing Infection

Patients cannot escape all manifestations of rheumatic disorders or side effects/complications of drugs, but they can avoid infection, one of the most frequent problems, in several ways. Clinicians should urge patients to:

1. Minimize exposure to cold—low temperatures reduce circulation and can cause tissue necrosis in the extremities. During cold weather, patients should wear warm socks, shoes, and gloves, as well as jackets and hats. When they must put their hands in a freezer, patients should work quickly and wear gloves if possible.
2. Avoid stressful situations—stress causes release of adrenaline, which causes vasoconstriction; this reduces the blood supply to the hands

and feet, which can lead to infection. Avoiding stress includes not driving during rush hours and taking lightly traveled routes at slower speeds whenever possible.

3. Treat wounds with great care—even slight scratches or bumps can damage taut, tender skin. Patients should wash broken skin, apply an antiseptic such as povidone iodine, and cover wounds with a sterile dressing. If they suffer a major laceration, they should have it treated by a physician.
4. Wash their hands frequently and thoroughly—the number of pathogens on hands can be reduced by washing the hands several times a day, from the nails up to the wrists. This is especially important before eating, after using bathroom facilities, and after handling possibly contaminated objects.

Eating Properly

Optimal nutrition is essential for everyone, yet this may be particularly difficult for chronically ill patients. Vitamin and mineral supplements can be helpful, but only as a supplement, not as a substitute for a balanced diet of protein, fresh fruits, and vegetables.

Claims that specific foods benefit patients with rheumatic diseases are seldom supported by scientific studies. One food of documented benefit is oily fish such as salmon and sardines; these contain epsilon-omega fatty acids that appear to decrease inflammation. Claims of vitamin and mineral supplements, advertised as particularly beneficial to rheumatic disease sufferers, must be regarded as speculative.

Clinicians should instruct patients to vary their diets, including foods from all basic groups. They should also remind patients that the following foods and products can be irritating to tender tissues: (1) highly acidic fruits (e.g., cranberries and plums) and vegetables (e.g., corn and lentils); (2) foods containing vinegar, spices, and hot pepper; (3) alcohol and tobacco; and (4) chewable vitamins (if vitamins are prescribed, they should be swallowed whole with 6 to 8 ounces of water).

Clinicians should instruct patients to vary their diets, including foods from all basic groups.

Clinicians should provide patients with ideas on how to prepare nutritious meals easily. These include: (1) chicken, which can be baked with white or sweet potatoes; (2) fish, which takes 3 minutes per pound to cook in a microwave oven; (3) vegetables, many of which take only 7 minutes per pound in a microwave oven; and (4) cottage cheese with fruit or sour cream, which takes almost no effort.

Exercising Appropriately

Following the baseline evaluations of a patient, a primary care physician or rheumatologist often refers the patient to a physical therapist who can design a personalized exercise program. Clinicians can also recommend that the patient, if an adult, participate in the Arthritis Foundation's "People with Arthritis Can Exercise (PACE®)" classes. Clinicians and patients should check with local chapters of the Arthritis Foundation to ascertain when 8-week PACE classes are scheduled.

Patients with rheumatic disorders, depending on the degree of their disabilities, can participate in any or all of three types of exercises:

1. Range of motion exercises involve moving joints gently as far as possible in all directions—to keep them from becoming stiff and deformed.
2. Strengthening exercises involve squeezing specific muscles tightly without moving the joint—to strengthen the muscles which support and move joints.
3. Aerobic exercises involve bringing the heart rate up to an optimal target level (computed according to the patient's age and physical condition) for 20 to 30 minutes. Because vigorous aerobic exercise classes can cause joint injury, patients should consider endurance exercises such as walking, swimming, or bicycling (regular or stationary bicycles), which do not put undue stress on their joints.[84]

Clinicians should provide patients with basic exercise guidelines. Patients with rheumatic disorders should:

1. Exercise when they have the least pain and stiffness (e.g., after a warm shower or after pharmacotherapy has taken effect)
2. Be consistent (e.g., do range of motion and strengthening exercises daily, and aerobic exercises 3 times per week)
3. Avoid rushing into an exercise program (i.e., start slowly, then gradually build up the routine)
4. Avoid overdoing exercises (i.e., the number of exercise repetitions to be performed depends on how a patient feels; too much exercise during a flare-up can exacerbate symptoms).
5. Wear proper shoes (e.g., well-cushioned athletic shoes, or custom-made shoes if disease has altered normal anatomy of feet).[84]

Participation in leisure activities (e.g., shuffleboard, golf, and gardening) also helps patients to avoid sedentary weight gain; these activities can be regulated to suit patients' abilities. Knitting, reading, writing, playing cards, and visiting with friends also keep the mind active and away from thoughts of food.

Alternative Therapies

Unless patients with rheumatic disorders understand the purpose of their treatment, they may become discouraged and turn to copper bracelets and mail-order potions. These useless nostrums often keep patients from continuing the effective medical therapy they need to manage their illnesses. Unfortunately, the fluctuations in disease activity, the limitations of available drugs, and the chronic nature of the disorders drive many patients to seek alternative treatments. Often, people forget that government agencies such as the Food and Drug Administration (FDA) carefully test drugs, devices, and interventions, under objective, rigorously-controlled conditions, for proof of efficacy. Those not approved—whether vitamins, herbal medicaments, or manipulations—have not been shown to help. Unfortunately, <u>lack</u> of governmental approval is often seen as a badge of honor, giving unproven remedies a cachet they would not otherwise have.

> Useless nostrums often keep patients from continuing the effective medical therapy they need to manage their diseases.

In fact, alternative treatments have grown into a multibillion dollar industry, prompting efforts by the National Institutes of Health and the American Academy of Sciences, among others, to re-evaluate everything from hypnosis to acupuncture to massage therapy. In certain situations, these and other nontraditional remedies may have a place in the treatment of rheumatic disorders. In general, however, such interventions should be considered adjuncts to, not substitutes for, pharmacotherapy and physical therapy. Further, patients should question their physicians about the availability of alternatives; many insurance companies now cover visits to chiropractors, acupuncturists, and nutritionists. These and other alternative approaches are likely to prove beneficial in the areas least responsive to traditional Western medicine, such as chronic pain, fatigue, and malaise, often with fewer side effects. On the other hand, patients should always be wary of outlandish claims and unfulfillable promises made by unlicensed practitioners of unapproved healing techniques.

Quality of Life

When patients understand the nature of their ailments, know their symptoms, and accept the periodic exacerbations, they are more inclined to make and keep appointments, and cooperate with their physicians. Patients should be knowledgeable about drugs they are taking (e.g., drug names, purposes, dosages, side effects). Clinicians should encourage patients to continue routine primary care, and stress the need for regular examinations and care to prevent medical and dental complications. Patients suffering morning stiffness should receive appointments in the late morning or the afternoon.

Patients who remain independent, adhere to a nutritionally sound diet, and continue to participate in normal social activities have the best chance of retaining or regaining positive self-images. Lack of mobility is the major hindrance to independence. Patients with rheumatic disorders sometimes lose the skill and confidence to drive safely. Clinicians should encourage them to use public transportation (buses, trains, taxis, etc.) when feasible, instead of relying on family members and friends for all their transportation needs. If patients' normal activities become too difficult for them, they should be told about the many aids and devices designed to help them perform simple tasks. (*See Chapter 8.*)

Chapter Summary

1. Clinicians can boost patients' morale by showing them concern, encouraging them to discuss their frustrations, and helping them to alleviate their pain and discomfort.
2. The simplest way to relieve pain is to apply cold or heat to the affected area, preferably under the guidance of a physical therapist.
3. Patients can relieve joint stress by: (1) maintaining normal weight and posture; (2) using ergometric aids; and (3) taking occasional breaks or changing position frequently when they must remain in one place for long periods.
4. During treatment, dental clinicians should give patients with rheumatic disorders frequent rest periods, and allow enough time for optimal therapy and patient comfort.
5. To avoid infection, patients should: (1) minimize exposure to cold; (2) avoid stressful situations; (3) treat wounds carefully; and (4) wash their hands frequently and thoroughly.
6. Clinicians should instruct patients to eat foods from all basic groups and to avoid foods and products which can irritate tender tissues.
7. Depending on the degree of their disabilities, patients with rheumatic disorders can participate in range of motion, strengthening, and/or aerobic exercises.
8. Useless nostrums often keep patients from continuing the effective medical therapy they need to manage their disorders.

Chapter 8 Useful Aids and Devices

Many items on the market are specifically designed to help the physically challenged. Other available articles, intended for general use, can make performing everyday tasks easier for the disabled. In addition, some common products can be altered or adapted to meet their needs.

The devices discussed in this chapter can be invaluable to patients with rheumatic disorders, and clinicians should tell patients about them. Clinicians should also ask patients about their own inventions and discoveries, to be shared with other patients. This tactic improves patients' self-esteem and clinicians' ability to deliver care and counseling.

Home Dental Care

Patients unable to lift their arms should lengthen their toothbrush handles (e.g., by taping tongue depressors to the handles or by cementing the handles inside a wooden cylinder).

Patients with limited hand closure, which prevents them from grasping or holding toothbrushes, can improve their ability to brush by:

1. Wrapping a Velcro strap, with a vinyl pocket designed to hold a toothbrush handle, around the hand
2. Taping a fingernail brush handle to a toothbrush
3. Inserting a toothbrush handle into a bicycle handle grip, or a Styrofoam™ or soft rubber ball.[94]

To use a power-assisted toothbrush safely, patients must be coordinated.

Other options include use of: (1) a special manual toothbrush called the Collis Curve, which brushes all exposed tooth surfaces simultaneously; and (2) a power-assisted toothbrush. However, to use a power-assisted toothbrush safely, patients must be coordinated; they must also be able to tolerate the brush's vibration and to operate the on/off mechanism. Patients can facilitate flossing by using plastic floss holders.[94]

Personal Comfort

When purchasing clothing and accessories, patients should choose:

1. Permanent press clothing, preferably with front openings and pockets
2. Well-designed running shoes which both cushion against impact and provide support for the feet (Shoes with Velcro closures are also helpful if patients have difficulty tying shoelaces.)
3. Handbags which can be carried over the shoulder.

Patients can purchase buttoning aids or make them by attaching a piece of wire to the end of a wooden handle. They can make zipper pulls by attaching a cup hook to a dowel rod.

For safety and comfort while bathing, patients suffering pain and loss of mobility should consider using:

1. Rails and seats that hook on the sides of bathtubs
2. Bath pillows, which support the head and shoulders
3. Rubber, nonslip grips in the tub
4. Long-handled bath brushes, to help in washing feet and back.

Drivers who cannot turn or move their heads without pain should look for special car seats and rear-view mirror extensions.

Meal Preparation

Patients whose fingers and hands lack strength and mobility should use lightweight, portable items for cooking and cleanup, and devices to help them function in the kitchen. These include:

1. Aluminum skillets with nonstick surfaces for stove-top cooking, instead of those made of stainless steel, glass, or cast iron
2. A microwave oven
3. Disposable aluminum pans, paper plates and cups, and plastic utensils
4. Electrically operated devices (e.g., an electric can opener, knife, food processor, blender, and small mixer with a pot scrubber attachment)
5. A pizza wheel, an electric knife, or an ergonomic knife, instead of a conventional knife
6. A jar opener which grips the lid, so the jar can be turned with both hands

7. A garbage can which opens with a foot pedal
8. A belt buckled to the refrigerator door as leverage to open the door with the forearm.

Housekeeping

Lightweight, portable items are also best for household chores; these include:

1. A child's mop and broom set, for dusting or for cleaning bathrooms
2. A mop with half the handle removed and 3 inches cut off the rags, for cleaning the tub or wiping up spills
3. Long-handled implements, for dusting furniture and reaching without straining
4. A cloth or towel placed over a doorknob, or a specially designed lever, making it easier to turn.

Further information on useful aids and devices for patients with rheumatic disorders can be obtained from the Arthritis Foundation. (*See listing in Appendix A.*)

Chapter Summary

1. Aids and devices which can assist physically challenged patients fall into three categories:
   a. Items specifically designed for these patients
   b. General use items
   c. Common products altered or adapted to meet physically challenged patients' needs.

2. Among the tasks which innovative aids and devices may facilitate are:
   a. Performing home dental care
   b. Dressing and bathing themselves
   c. Preparing meals
   d. Doing household chores.

Progress Test G

1. When patients' abilities to perform routine tasks are affected by rheumatic diseases/syndromes, their ______________ __ ___________ suffers.

2. To relieve pain caused by an acute inflammatory reaction, patients should apply _______ to the affected area; to relieve chronic pain, patients should apply _______ to the affected area, unless they have decreased sensation or circulation or a sensitivity to _______.

3. Patients should continue their pharmacotherapy as prescribed, even during periods of ______________ ______________.

4. ___________ places stress on all weight-bearing joints; _______ _____________ puts stress on the spine, neck and shoulders.

5. When patients suffer acute TMJ pain, ___________________ dental treatment should be postponed.

6. Adrenaline released during stressful situations causes ____________________, reducing the blood supply to the hands and feet, which can lead to infection.

7. Highly acidic fruits, which can irritate tender tissues, include plums and ____________________.

8. ______________ exercises involve bringing the heart rate up to an optimal target level for 20 to 30 minutes.

9. Instead of using a conventional knife when cooking or eating, patients with rheumatic disorders may find it easier to use a pizza wheel, or an electric or _________________ knife.

Answers to Progress Tests

Test A (Chapter 1)

1. 30, 60
2. synovium
3. support
4. slowly, insidiously
5. more prolonged
6. nails, thumbs
7. ankylosis
8. inflamed joints
9. 2 years
10. NSAIDs, DMARD

Test B (Chapter 2)

1. inflammation
2. criteria
3. diagnostic tool
4. severe fatigue
5. viral-like
6. delta wave sleep
7. tender points
8. sleep apnea
9. irritable bowel
10. pharmacotherapy, nondrug

Test C (Chapter 3)

1. skin, organ
2. autoantibodies
3. rise, fall
4. cutaneous, mucosal
5. malar, nasolabial
6. discoid, alopecia
7. thrombocytopenia
8. swan neck
9. causes of death
10. natural, artificial

Test D (Chapter 4)

1. salivary, lacrimal
2. multiple
3. foamy saliva
4. sandy, gritty
5. parched, burning
6. Raynaud's phenomenon
7. bromhexine
8. recurrent caries
9. malnutrition
10. extreme care

Test E (Chapter 5)

1. limited, diffuse
2. 40, 60
3. proximal
4. diffuse
5. Calcinosis
6. arteriolar spasm
7. peristalsis
8. muscle exercises
9. Blood pressure
10. an hour or more

Test F (Chapter 6)

1. myelosuppression
2. cyclophosphamide
3. 20 weeks
4. Amsler
5. MTX
6. fetal kernicterus
7. cholesterol, smoking
8. salicylates, aspirin
9. misoprostol
10. Tricyclic antidepressants

Test G (Chapters 7 and 8)

1. standard of living
2. cold, heat, heat
3. relative comfort
4. Obesity, poor posture
5. nonemergency
6. vasoconstriction
7. cranberries
8. Aerobic
9. ergonomic

Definitions, Abbreviations, & Acronyms

ACE inhibitor — a drug used to treat hypertension by inhibiting reactions of the angiotensin-converting enzyme. *See Angiotensin.*
Acinar — pertaining to an acinus, one of many small sac-like parts found in a compound gland.
ACR — American College of Rheumatology.
Acupuncture — a method of inserting sharp, fine needles into specific points on the body, to relieve pain or anesthetize certain areas.
Acute — pertaining to a process (symptom, condition, or disease) having a rapid onset, severe symptoms, and a short course.
Adenopathy — glandular enlargement, especially of the lymph nodes.
Agranulocytosis — an acute disease, possibly the result of drugs or radiation, which produces high fever and a rapid drop in circulating granular white blood cells.
Alopecia — baldness; hair loss.
Amyloid — an abnormal protein-polysaccharide having starch-like characteristics and associated with a number of chronic diseases such as multiple myeloma, tuberculosis, Hodgkin's disease, and carcinoma.
ANA — antinuclear antibody.
Analgesic — (1) relieving pain; (2) an agent that relieves pain without causing loss of consciousness.
Anaphylaxis (literally, "without protection") — an immediate, well-defined, antigen-antibody reaction to an allergen (e.g., a specific food or drug).
Angiotensin — a vasopressing polypeptide found in the blood.
Angular cheilitis — inflammation and cracks at the corners of the lips.
Ankylosis — joint immobility caused by injury, disease, or surgery.
Anorexia nervosa — an eating disorder in which patients refuse to maintain a normal body weight, are afraid of gaining weight, and have distorted perceptions of their body shapes or sizes.
Anti-dsDNA — antibody to double-stranded DNA. *See Appendix B, Table 9.*
Anti-La/SS-B — antibody to La/SS-B. *See Appendix B, Table 9.*
Anti-Ro/SS-A — antibody to Ro/SS-A. *See Appendix B, Table 9.*
Anti-Sm — antibody to a small ribonucleoprotein (SmRNP). *See Appendix B, Table 9.*
Antibody — one of many immunoglobulins (protein molecules), manufactured by the lymphocytes, which function as a primary immune defense; each antibody neutralizes or destroys a specific antigen (foreign protein).
Antigen — a substance, such as a toxin, foreign protein, bacterium, or cell tissue, capable of inducing an immune response (i.e., stimulating production of an antibody).
Antinuclear antibody (ANA) — an autoantibody to the nuclear portion of cells.
Antiphospholipid syndrome — a group of disorders which can include thrombosis (arterial and venous), thrombocytopenia, spontaneous abortions, and pulmonary hypertension.
Aortitis — inflammation of the aorta.
Aplastic anemia (also: pancytopenia) — a form of anemia in which the bone marrow's ability to generate red blood cells is deficient; may be caused by bone marrow disease or exposure to toxic substances. *See also Bone marrow.*
ARA — American Rheumatism Association; former name of ACR.
Arrhythmia — irregular or abnormal rhythm of the heart beat.
Arteriole (adj. arteriolar) — a very small arterial branch, especially one adjacent to a capillary.
Arthralgia — pain in a joint. *See Polyarthralgia.*
Arthritis (pl. arthritides) — inflammation of a joint, usually accompanied by pain, swelling, warmth, and redness. *See also Nonerosive arthritis.*
Arthrocentesis — *See Appendix B, Table 10.*
Arthroplasty — an operation to reconstruct or reshape a diseased joint.

Articular — pertaining to a joint. *See Extraarticular.*
Articulate — consisting of sections which unite to form a joint.
Articulation — the place of junction (or union) between skeletal bones.
AST — aspartate aminotransferase.
Ataxia — defective voluntary muscular coordination.
Atherogenesis — the formation of atheromatous lesions (plaque) in the walls of arteries.
Atherosclerosis — a common form of arteriosclerosis in which yellowish cholesterol-containing plaques form within arteries.
Atrophy — a wasting away, deterioration, or shrinkage, especially of a cell, tissue, organ, or body part.
Autoantibody — an antibody (immunoglobulin) that an organism produces to combat any of its own components.
Autoimmunity — a condition characterized by an immune response to the body's own tissues.
AZA — azathioprine.
Bartholin's gland — a small mucous gland in the lateral wall of the vaginal vestibule; also called glandula vestibularis major.
Biofeedback — the use of devices which provide information on such bodily functions as blood pressure or heart rate, helping patients to exert some voluntary control over those functions.
Bipolar disorders — a group of mood disorders, most of which cause manic, depressive, or mixed episodes, sometimes with psychotic or melancholic features.
Blood serum — the clear liquid which separates from completely clotted blood.
Bone marrow — the red or yellow, soft, fatty tissue found in bone cavities. Red bone marrow is blood-producing tissue, gradually replaced in some bones, as the body ages, by less active yellow marrow.
Bouchard's node — a bony enlargement of the proximal interphalangeal (PIP) joint.
Bulimia nervosa — an eating disorder characterized by eating binges and, in many cases, purging to avoid the consequences.
Calcinosis — abnormal deposition of calcium salts in body tissues.
Candidiasis — an infection of moist cutaneous areas of the body, caused by the yeast-like fungus *Candida albicans*.
Carditis — inflammation of the heart.
Caries, dental — tooth decay; usually involves gradual disintegration of calcified tissue on a tooth surface.
Carpal tunnel syndrome — a group of symptoms caused by the compression of the median nerve as it enters the palm; symptoms include pain, tingling, and numbness in the fingers and hand, sometimes extending to the elbow.
Cartilage — a resilient connective tissue comprising part of the skeleton (e.g., it covers the articular surfaces of bones, preventing them from rubbing against each other).
CBC — complete blood cell count.
Cellulitis —an infection of subcutaneous or deeper tissues, resulting in acute, diffuse, edematous, and suppurative inflammation.
Cervical — pertaining to the neck or the cervix.
Charley horse — pain and stiffness in a muscle, usually the thigh quadriceps, caused by a strain or tear.
Chilblain — a recurrent, localized, painful itching and swelling on fingers, toes, or ears; caused by exposure to damp cold.
Cholinergic — activated by or able to free acetylcholine (e.g., the nerve fibers in the parasympathetic nervous system, the craniosacral division of the autonomic nervous system).
Chronic — pertaining to a process (symptom, condition, or disease) having a long course or recurring frequently.
CNS — central nervous system.
Cock-up toe deformity — an MTP joint change caused by RA; characterized by upward dislocation of a proximal phalange on a metatarsal head.
Cognition (adj. cognitive) — the mental process of knowing, including such things as awareness, perception, judgment, and reasoning.
Collagen — the fibrous protein constituent of bone, tendons, cartilage, and connective tissue.
Coma — deep unconsciousness, often prolonged; usually resulting from injury, disease, or use of drugs.
Complement system — a group of over 20 proteins in the blood serum which react with antibodies and then interact to cause inflammation; low complement levels indicate active disease. *See Appendix B, Table 9.*

Complication — a secondary disease or accident occurring during the course of another but not necessarily related, yet affecting the course of the original ailment.
Condyle (adj. condylar) — a rounded protuberance on a bone, usually one that is part of an articulation.
Conjunctivitis — inflammation of the conjunctiva, the mucous membrane lining the eyelids and covering the forepart of the sclera (the white outer coat of the eyeball).
Connective tissue — a type of tissue which supports and/or connects other tissues and body parts.
Contracture — joint or muscle immobility caused by fibrosis of the supporting connective tissue. *See also Flexion contracture.*
Crepitus — a dry or crackling sound.
CRP — C-reactive protein. *See Appendix B, Table 9.*
Crust — an outer layer of solid matter formed by the drying of exudate or secretions.
Cutaneous — pertaining to the skin.
Cyanosis (adj. cyanotic) — bluish discoloration of skin due to reduced hemoglobin level in the blood.
Cytokine — an intercellular mediator of immune responses.
Cytotoxic — pertaining to an agent which has a specific destructive effect on certain cells.
Delusional disorder — a state in which a patient holds a false belief or makes an inaccurate inference about external reality, contrary to what everybody else believes and what is objectively proved.
Dementia — a general loss of intellectual abilities, including memory, judgment, and abstract thinking.
Deoxyribonucleic acid (DNA) — the main constituent of a cell's chromosomes; in all organisms except RNA viruses, it contains the genetic code. *See RNA.*
Depression, mental — a condition marked by deep sadness and lack of any pleasurable interest in life.
Dermatitis — inflammation of the skin.
Dermatomyositis — a collagen disease marked by inflammation of the skin, subcutaneous tissue, and muscles, and necrosis of muscle fibers.
Digit — a finger or a toe.
DIP — distal interphalangeal.
Disease — a pathologic bodily state exhibiting a group of specific clinical signs and symptoms, with laboratory findings exclusive to it; these differentiate the condition from other normal or abnormal states. Disease is distinct from illness in that the former is generally tangible and measurable, whereas the latter is usually subjective (e.g., pain or malaise).
Discoid — disk-shaped.
Disorder — a mental or physical abnormality.
DNA — deoxyribonucleic acid.
Dyspareunia — pain in vaginolabial areas during or after sexual intercourse.
Dyspepsia — painful or imperfect digestion, symptomatic of other disorders.
Dysphagia — inability to swallow or difficulty in swallowing.
Dyspnea — difficulty in breathing, especially shortness of breath.
EBV — Epstein-Barr virus.
Ecchymosis —a small hemorrhagic spot, larger than a petechia, in the skin or mucous membrane, forming a nonelevated, rounded or irregular, blue or purplish patch.
Edema (adj. edematous) — an excessive accumulation of fluid in tissue spaces.
Effusion — escape of fluid into a cavity, tissue, or other body part. *See also Synovial effusion.*
Electrocardiogram (EKG) — a graphic tracing of variations in electrical potentials of the heart muscle and cardiac nerves.
Electroencephalogram (EEG) — a recording of the brain's electrical activity; variations in EEG patterns correlate well with activity and conditions in the brain.
Embolus (pl. emboli) — a clot of undissolved matter which blood or lymph current has brought from a larger blood vessel to a smaller one, where it may obstruct blood circulation.
Endocarditis — an inflammation of and irregular growths on the membrane which lines the heart cavities and forms its valves.
Endothelium (adj. endothelial) — a layer of epithelial cells lining the heart cavities, the serous cavities, and the lymphatic and blood vessels.
Enthesopathy — an ailment involving the bony attachment of muscles or tendons.
Epicondyle — an eminence above the condyle on a bone.
Epithelium (adj. epithelial) — the tissue that covers internal and external body surfaces, vessels, and small cavities.
Epstein-Barr virus — infectious mononucleosis.

Ergometric — pertaining to something which reduces fatigue and discomfort.
Erosion — an eating or gnawing away (e.g., in RA, a wearing away of cartilage or bone by synovitis); a shallow or superficial ulceration.
Erythema (adj. erythematous) — abnormal redness of the skin or mucous membrane, produced by capillary congestion.
ESR — erythrocyte sedimentation rate. *See Appendix B, Table 9.*
Etiology — the science dealing with causes of disease.
Exocrine gland — a gland whose secretions, after flowing through a duct, lubricate the skin or mucous membranes.
Extensor — a muscle which extends a joint.
Extraarticular — occurring or situated outside a joint.
Fibrin — an insoluble protein essential to clotting of blood, formed by action of thrombin on fibrinogen.
Fibroblast — an immature, fiber-producing connective tissue cell.
Fibrosis — the formation of fibrous tissue, as in a reparative or reactive process, in excessive amounts.
Fibular deviation — an MTP joint change caused by chronic synovitis; characterized by deviation of the toes in a fibular direction with respect to the metatarsals.
Fissure — a cleft or groove.
Flexion contracture — a joint deformity characterized by the inability to be bent. *See Contracture.*
Follicular — in the hair follicles of the skin.
Gastric — pertaining to, affecting, or originating in the stomach.
Gastrointestinal — pertaining to the stomach and intestines.
GI tract — gastrointestinal tract; the stomach and intestines in continuity.
Glaucoma — one of several eye diseases characterized by intraocular pressure, optic nerve atrophy, and various degrees of vision loss.
Glomerulonephritis — a form of nephritis characterized by lesions primarily affecting the glomeruli, clustered capillary blood vessels in the kidneys.
Glossitis — inflammation of the tongue.
Glucose 6-phosphate dehydrogenase (G6PD) — an intermediate in carbohydrate metabolism.
Goodpasture's syndrome — glomerulonephritis accompanied by pulmonary hemorrhage and other adverse conditions.
Gout — an inflammatory, arthritic condition characterized by uric acid crystal deposits in joint spaces.
HCQ — hydroxychloroquine.
Heberden's node — a bony enlargement of the distal interphalangeal (DIP) joint.
Hematocrit (HCT) — (1) the volume of mature red blood cells (erythrocytes), packed by centrifugation, in a given volume of blood; (2) a marked tube used in a centrifuge to determine HCT.
Hematologic — pertaining to the blood and blood-forming tissues.
Hemoglobin (HGB) — the iron-containing pigment of red blood cells; HGB carries oxygen from the lungs to the tissues.
Hemolytic — pertaining to, characterized by, or producing disruption of the integrity of red blood cell membranes, causing release of hemoglobin.
Hepatic — pertaining to the liver.
Hepatitis — an inflammation of the liver, caused by viruses or other toxins.
Hepatomegaly — enlargement of the liver.
Hepatosplenomegaly — an enlarged liver and spleen.
Histocompatibility locus antigen — an antigen located on all the body's nucleated cells, which identifies a cell as self, and is important in controlling the magnitude and presence of antibody responses.
Histopathology (adj. histopathologic) — the study of microscopic tissue changes caused by disease.
HLA — histocompatibility locus antigen.
Hyperemia — excessive blood flow to a body part.
Hyperplasia (adj. hyperplastic) — an abnormal increase or multiplication in the number of cells.
Hyperreninemia — increased renin (an enzyme produced by the kidney) in blood, associated with hypertension.
Hypermobility — excessive movement (e.g., joint instability).
Hypertension — abnormally or chronically high blood pressure; a major symptom of arterial disease.
Hypertrophy — increased organ size, without tumor formation.
Hypoglycemia — abnormally low concentration of blood glucose.

Hypomobility — diminished movement (e.g., of joints).
Hypomotility (also: hypokinesia) — decreased motor reaction to stimulus (e.g., esophageal hypomotility).
Hypopigmentation — abnormally diminished pigmentation.
Hypotensive reaction — a drop in blood pressure due to an outside stimulus.
Hypotension — abnormally low blood pressure.
Hypothyroidism — abnormally low thyroid secretion, causing a lowered basal metabolic rate.
Iatrogenic — unforeseen or unintended effect of treatment.
Idiopathic — referring to a disease which has no known cause.
Immunoglobulin — one of a family of proteins (designated IgA, IgD, IgE, IgG, and IgM), many of which function as antibodies but lack antigen specificity. All antibodies are immunoglobulins.
Immunosuppressant — a drug which inhibits the normal immune response.
Immunosuppressive — capable of inhibiting the normal immune response; drugs, surgery, or diseases can do this.
Indurated — hardened; abnormally hard.
Infarct — an area of tissue dying because of an obstructed blood supply.
Interleukin — a protein substance, produced by macrophages and other cells, which induces helper T-cells to produce interleukin-2 and stimulate inflammatory responses.
Interstitial — pertaining to spaces within an organ.
Interstitial cystitis — inflammation of the bladder wall.
Interstitial lung disease — a group of disorders of the lower respiratory tract, primarily affecting the alveolar wall structures; SSc patients with this disorder may develop irreversible interstitial pulmonary fibrosis. *See Fibrosis.*
Intraarticular — within a joint.
Iridocyclitis — inflammation of the iris and the structure directly behind it (the ciliary body).
Irritable bowel syndrome — a chronic disease characterized by cramping and altered bowel habits (noninflammatory diarrhea or constipation, or both); may be initiated or exacerbated by stress.
Ischemia — deficient blood supply to a body part, caused by obstruction of blood circulation.
Jaundice — yellowing of the skin and other tissues, caused by bile pigment deposition due to excess bilirubin in circulation.
Joint — *see Articulation.*
Juxtaarticular — situated close to a joint.
KCS — keratoconjunctivitis sicca.
Keratitis — inflammation of the cornea.
Keratoconjunctivitis sicca — an eye disorder characterized by hyperemia of the conjunctiva due to a deficiency of tears; possible thickening of the cornea and impaired visual acuity.
Kernicterus (also bilirubin encephalopathy) — a condition associated with abnormally high bilirubin levels in the blood; characterized by severe, destructive neural changes.
Lacrimal gland — one of the glands which secretes tears to lubricate the eyes.
LE — lupus erythematosus.
Leukocyte — any colorless, ameboid cell mass, especially a white blood cell; also a pus or lymph corpuscle, or wandering connective tissue cell.
Leukocytosis — an abnormal number of white blood cells; a transient condition.
Leukopenia — reduction in the number of leukocytes in the blood.
Lichen planus — an inflammatory disease of the skin and mucosa; the lesion consists of red to violet papules covered with a fine white scale.
Livedo reticularis — a mottled skin discoloration caused by small vessel vasculitis.
Lymphadenopathy — diseased lymph nodes.
Lymphocyte — a mononuclear, nonphagocytic leukocyte crucial to the adaptive part of the immune system, which mounts a tailor-made defense when invading pathogens penetrate the body's general defenses, such as those provided by other types of white blood cells.
Lymphoma — any of a group of cancers in which lymphoid tissue cells multiply unchecked.
Lymphopenia — decrease in the number of lymphocytes in the blood.
Macule — a small (<1 cm) discolored spot, level with the skin's surface; an area distinguishable by color from its surroundings. If >1 cm, it is called a patch.
Malaise — a feeling of bodily discomfort or uneasiness, often indicative of infection or other illness.
Malar — pertaining to the cheek.
Malocclusion — malposition and imperfect contact of the teeth of the upper and lower jaws.

Mandibular — pertaining to the lower jaw.
Manifestation — the demonstrable presence of a sign or symptom associated with a specific disease/syndrome.
MCP — metacarpophalangeal.
Melancholy (adj. melancholic) — a state in which an individual loses interest or pleasure in most or all activities or fails to react to usually pleasurable stimuli.
Micrognathia — an abnormally small jaw, especially the lower jaw.
Mitral stenosis — an abnormal narrowing or contracting of the mitral valve within the heart.
Mitral valve prolapse — prolapse (falling or slipping out of place) of the left atrioventricular valve, located between the left ventricle and left atrium of the heart.
MTP — metatarsophalangeal.
MTX — methotrexate.
Mucolytic — an agent which dissolves or destroys mucin, the chief constituent of mucus.
Mucous membrane — a mucus-secreting membrane lining all bodily passages open to the air (e.g., parts of the digestive and respiratory tracts).
Multiple sclerosis — a CNS disease in which infiltrating lymphocytes degrade the myelin sheath of nerves.
Myalgia — muscular pain or tenderness.
Myasthenia gravis — a disorder characterized by weakness of the skeletal muscles and worsening fatigue.
Myeloma — a tumor composed of bone marrow cells.
Myelosuppression — suppressed bone marrow activity, causing a reduction in platelets, white cells, and red cells. *See also Bone marrow.*
Myocarditis — inflammation of the middle, thickest layer of the heart wall, composed of cardiac muscle.
Myocardium (adj. myocardial) — the middle, thickest muscle layer of the heart wall.
Myopathy —inflammation of striated muscle tissue; caused by infection or adverse reaction to a drug.
Myopericarditis — combined inflammation of the myocardium and pericardium.
Nail fold — the groove in skin surrounding the margins and proximal edges of a fingernail or toenail.
Necrosis (adj. necrotic) — death of a cell or of a group of cells in contact with living tissue; caused by the progressive degradation of enzyme action.
Necrotizing vasculitis (also: necrotizing angiitis) — a disorder characterized by blood vessel inflammation and necrosis.
Nephritis — inflammation of the kidney. *See Glomerulonephritis.*
Neuritis — inflammation of the peripheral nerves.
Neurologic — pertaining to the nervous system.
Neurotransmitter — a neuron-released chemical substance ("chemical messenger") which crosses a synapse to bind to a receptor on an adjacent neuron. *See Synapse.*
Neutropenia — an abnormally small number of neutrophil cells (granulocytic white cells) in the blood.
Nodule — a small, solid lump detectable by touch.
Nonerosive arthritis — inflammation of the joints which does not cause tissue destruction.
Nosologic — pertaining to nosology, the classification of diseases.
Nostrum — a quack, patent, or secret remedy, untested and of unproved effectiveness.
NSAID — nonsteroidal anti-inflammatory drug.
Nystagmus — involuntary, rapid eyeball movement.
Occular — pertaining to the eye or vision.
Occult blood — feces blood, detectable only by microscopic or spectroscopic examination or by a chemical test; indicates internal bleeding.
Opacification — a condition rendering the cornea impenetrable by light.
Organic brain syndrome — a group of mental disorders associated with brain damage impairing cerebral function.
Osteoporosis — abnormal, progressive rarefaction of bone; bones break easily and heal slowly; the disease may be idiopathic or occur secondarily to other diseases.
Palpation — the process of examining or exploring by touching.
Pancreatitis — inflammation of the pancreas.
Pannus — invasion of a joint by richly perfused inflammatory tissue.
Papule — a small (<1 cm), circumscribed, solid, elevated lesion of the skin.

Paresthesia — a skin sensation, e.g., burning, prickling, tingling, or itching, with no apparent physical cause.
Parotid gland — one of a pair of salivary glands situated on the face, below and in front of the ears.
Parotitis — inflammation of a parotid gland.
Pathogen — a microbe (bacterium, virus, fungus, parasitic protozoan) that can infect a susceptible host and cause a disease.
Pericarditis — inflammation of the fibroserous sac enclosing the heart and the roots of the great blood vessels.
Pericardium (adj. pericardial) — the fluid-filled membranous sac surrounding the heart.
Periosteum (adj. periosteal) — a specialized connective tissue covering all bones and having bone-forming potential.
Peripheral neuropathy — diseases and disorders affecting the nerves that fan out from the CNS to the muscles, skin, internal organs, and glands.
Peristalsis — progressive waves of involuntary muscle contractions and relaxations that move matter along certain tube-like structures of the body, especially the alimentary canal.
Peritonitis — inflammation of the serous membrane lining the walls of the abdominal and pelvic cavities.
Periungual — around a fingernail or toenail.
Petechia (pl. petechiae) — a small red spot on the skin or a mucous or serous membrane, caused by a minute hemorrhage.
Phagocyte (adj. phagocytic) — a cell which ingests waste material, harmful bacteria, etc., in the tissues and bloodstream.
Photosensitivity — an abnormal cutaneous response to natural and/or artificial ultraviolet light, and to unshielded, white fluorescent light.
Pigmentation — the deposit of coloring matter; the coloration or discoloration of tissue by a pigment.
PIP — proximal interphalangeal.
Plaque — a small, raised, disk-shaped formation or growth >1 cm; a patch.
Plasmapheresis — injection of red blood cells rather than whole blood.
Pleura (adj. pleural) — the serous membrane which enfolds the lungs and lines the chest cavity walls.
Pleurisy/pleuritis — inflammation of the pleura.
Pneumonitis — inflammation of the lung tissue.
Polyarthralgia — pain in several joints.
Polyarthritis — inflammation of several joints.
Polymyalgia rheumatica — a poorly understood disorder characterized by shoulder and pelvic girdle pain, abnormally high ESR, and morning stiffness; frequently affects women >50 years of age.
Polymyositis — a necrotizing disease of striated muscle tissue.
Polyuria — excessive and/or frequent urination, as in cases of diabetes.
Prophylactic — a drug, procedure, or type of equipment used to prevent disease.
Prostatitis — inflammation of the prostate gland.
Proteinuria — excess serum proteins in the urine.
Pruritus (adj. pruritic) — itchiness.
Psoriasis — a chronic skin disease, characterized by erythematous papules forming plaques with distinct borders.
Psychosis (adj. psychotic) — historically, this term has been applied to many disorders; in general, it can be defined as clinically significant impairment of mental functioning which prevents a sufferer from meeting the ordinary demands of life; characterized by delusions, hallucinations, agitation, disorganization, and/or incoherent speech, with no awareness on the part of the patient that this behavior is abnormal.
Pulmonary hypertension — abnormally high blood pressure within the lungs.
Purpura — purple or red-brown skin lesions, caused by the degradation of blood that has pooled after its escape from blood vessels and/or capillaries damaged by disease or trauma.
RA — rheumatoid arthritis.
Renal — pertaining to the kidneys.
Reticulocytosis — an abnormally high number of reticulocytes (young red cells) in peripheral blood.
RF — rheumatoid factor.
Rheumatic disease — a general term for a disease marked by inflammation and/or pain in muscles and/or joints.

Rheumatism (adj. rheumatic) — any acute or chronic condition characterized by inflammation, muscle soreness and stiffness, and/or joint pain (e.g., arthritis, degenerative joint disease, bursitis, fibromyositis, etc.).
Rheumatoid factor — an immunoglobulin autoantibody often found in the blood serum of patients with RA and Sjögren's.
Rhinitis — inflammation of the nasal mucous membranes.
Ribonucleic acid — a nucleic acid that contains genetic instructions for the synthesis of proteins.
RNA — ribonucleic acid.
Rub — the sound of friction when serous surfaces move against each other.
Sacroiliitis — inflammation of the sacroiliac joint.
Sarcoidosis — a disease, origin unknown, which causes granulomatous lesions to form, especially in the skin, lungs, liver, and lymph nodes.
Scale — a thin, flaky, compacted layer of epithelial cells on the body surface.
Scapula spine — a triangular bone plate, one edge of which is attached to the back of the scapula.
Schirmer test — *see Appendix B, Table 10.*
Schizophrenia — a psychotic disorder, lasting at least 6 months, in which the patient has at least two of the following symptoms: delusions, hallucinations, disorganized speech, greatly disorganized or catatonic behavior.
Scintigraphy — *see Appendix B, Table 10.*
Scleritis — inflammation of the sclera, the tissue covering the "white" of the eye.
Sclerodactyly (or acrosclerosis) — localized induration and tightening of the skin (e.g., of the digits and face) caused by SSc.
Sclerosis — an induration (hardening) of tissue or an organ, especially when caused by fibrosis.
Seizure — a sudden episode of uncontrolled electrical activity in the brain.
Self-tolerance — no immune response to one's own antigens.
Serositis — inflammation of a serous membrane.
Serotonin — a chemical (5-hydroxytryptamine) present in many body tissues; in the CNS, it inhibits neurotransmission.
Serous — producing, resembling, or containing serum (e.g., a membrane which lines a serous cavity).
Serum — the clear portion of any body liquid, especially the fluid moistening the surface of serous membranes. *See also: Blood serum.*
Sialography — *see Appendix B, Table 10.*
Side effect — the secondary action of a drug, often undesirable.
Sign — an objective indication of disease, especially observable physical, radiologic, and laboratory evidence.
SLE — systemic lupus erythematosus.
Sleep apnea — cessation of breathing during sleep; to be classified as sleep apnea, the cessation of breathing should last at least 10 seconds and occur ≥30 times during a 7-hour period of sleep.
Somatic — referring to the body as a whole, rather than to a specific body part or the mind.
Somatoform disorder — a group of mental disorders characterized by physical symptoms suggesting a medical condition but not fully explained by the presence of a medical condition, the direct effects of a substance (e.g., a drug), or another mental disorder.
Splenomegaly — enlargement of the spleen.
Spirometer —a instrument used to measure the amount of air inhaled into and exhaled from the lungs.
Spondylitis — inflammation of one or more vertebrae.
SS — Sjögren's syndrome.
SSZ — sulfasalazine.
Stomatitis — inflammation of oral mucous tissues.
Subacute — somewhat acute; between acute and chronic.
Subchondral — beneath a cartilage.
Subcutaneous — beneath the skin.
Subluxation — incomplete or partial dislocation.
Suppurate — to produce pus.
Swan-neck deformity — a sign of RA characterized by flexion contracture of the MCP joints, hyperextension of the PIP joints, and flexion of the DIP joints.
Swelling — an abnormal enlargement, anywhere on or in the body, usually temporary (e.g., swelling caused by metabolic disturbance, trauma, or infection).

Sydenham's chorea — a childhood disease characterized by involuntary, purposeless muscle contractions, memory impairment, and anxiety.
Symptom — a subjective indication of disease, especially a patient's report of an abnormal physical or emotional condition.
Synapse — the microscopic gap between any two neurons.
Syndrome — a group of symptoms and/or signs which together are characteristic of a specific disease or disorder.
Synovia (also: synovial fluid) — the lubricating fluid secreted by the synovium of a joint, bursa, or tendon sheath.
Synovial — pertaining to synovia.
Synovial effusion — an increase of synovia in the joint capsule.
Synovial joint — a joint separated by space containing synovia, which permits more or less free movement.
Synovitis — inflammation of a synovium.
Synovium (also: synovial membrane) — the inner layer of a joint capsule's surface.
Systemic — affecting or pertaining to the whole body.
Tarsal tunnel syndrome — a group of symptoms, including pain in and numbness of the sole of the foot, caused by pressure on the tibial nerve as it passes through the tarsal tunnel.
Telangiectasia — a vascular lesion formed by dilation of a group of small blood vessels. Characteristically, a telangiectatic or spider lesion is red in the center, with red tendrils or legs running out from it.
Tendon — a strong band of fibrous tissue which connects muscle to bone.
Thrombocytopenia — a diminished blood platelet count.
Thrombosis — the presence or formation of a blood clot (thrombus) within the vascular system.
Thyroxine — a subnormal level of serum thyroxine indicates hypothyroidism; an abnormally high level indicates hyperthyroidism.
Thyroid stimulating hormone (TSH) — a subnormal level of serum TSH indicates hyperthyroidism.
Tinnitus — a noise in the ears (e.g., ringing, roaring, buzzing, clicking), not caused by an outside source but, usually, by a disease, injury, blockage, or drug.
Titer — the degree to which a substance may be diluted before it loses its ability to react with another substance. The term is generally associated with measurement of serum antibody levels.
Topical — pertaining to a definite, or local, area.
Trauma — (1) an injury caused by an extrinsic agent; (2) a disordered psychologic state resulting from physical injury or stress.
Tumor — (1) swelling, one of the cardinal signs of inflammation; morbid enlargement; (2) neoplasm; a new growth of tissue in which cell multiplication is uncontrolled and progressive.
Tumor necrosis factor — a cytokine released by macrophages which can cause in vivo hemorrhagic necrosis of some tumor cells.
Ulcer — a local defect or excavation of the surface of an organ or tissue, produced by the sloughing of necrotic inflammatory tissue.
Ulnar deviation — an MCP joint change caused by chronic synovitis; characterized by deviation of the long axis of the fingers in an ulnar direction with respect to the metacarpals.
Uremia — the retention of excessive by-products of protein metabolism in the blood, and the toxic condition produced thereby, marked by nausea, vomiting, vertigo, convulsions, and coma; usually due to abnormal renal function.
Urethritis — inflammation of the urethra.
Urticaria (also: hives) — a skin eruption of very itchy wheals, caused by an allergy, an infection, or a nervous reaction.
Uveitis — a nonspecific, intraocular inflammation.
Vascular — pertaining to blood vessels.
Vascularization — development of new blood vessels, especially abnormal or pathologic blood vessels.
Vasculitis (adj. vasculitic)— inflammation of a blood vessel. *See also Necrotizing vasculitis.*
Vasoconstrictor an agent causing narrowing of the blood vessels.
Vasodilator — an agent causing an increase in the diameter of blood vessels.
Visceral — pertaining to a viscus (any large thoracic or abdominal organ).
Vulvodynia — a syndrome with no known cause, characterized by vulval itching, discomfort, and pain, especially during sexual intercourse.

Appendix A Selected Resources

RHEUMATOID ARTHRITIS

American College of Rheumatology (ACR)
60 Executive Park South, Ste. 150
Atlanta, GA 30329
1-404-633-3777
Publication: journal—*Arthritis & Rheumatism*

Arthritis Foundation
1330 W. Peachtree St., Atlanta, GA 30309
P.O. Box 7669, Atlanta, GA 30357-0669
1-800-283-7800; information: 1-800-207-8633;
membership: 1-800-933-0032 or 1-404-872-7100
Internet: www.arthritis.org
150 local offices in the United States
Offers: Arthritis Self-Help Course; People With Arthritis Can Exercise (PACE®) classes.
Publications: nontechnical leaflets describing various rheumatic disorders—for patients; *Primer on the Rheumatic Diseases* and many other technical publications—for clinicians

National Institute of Arthritis and Musculoskeletal and Skin Diseases
National Institutes of Health
1 AMS Circle, Bethesda, MD 20892-3675
1-301-496-8188
Coordinates federal research on rheumatic diseases

CHRONIC FATIGUE AND FIBROMYALGIA SYNDROMES

American Assoc. for Chronic Fatigue Syndrome (AACFS)
7 Van Buren St., Albany, NY 12206
1-518-482-2202; 1-800-232-8710
fax 518-435-1765
Offers: packet for clinicians

CFIDS Association of America, Inc.
P.O. Box 220398, Charlotte, NC 28222-0398
1-800-442-3437 or 1-900-988-2343
Offers: patient education and support

CFS/ME Computer Networking Project
For information, e-mail request to:
cfs-me@sjuvm,stjohns.edu.

Fibromyalgia Network
P.O. Box 31750, Tucson, AZ 85751-1750
1-520-290-5508; 1-800-853-2929
Offers: patient education and referrals to support groups in all states

National Chronic Fatigue Syndrome and Fibromyalgia Association (NCFSFA)
3521 Broadway, Ste. 222, Kansas City, MO 64111
1-816-931-4777
Offers: patient education and support

CLINICAL PRODUCTS LISTS

American Dental Association
211 E. Chicago Ave., Chicago, IL 60611
1-312-440-2500.
Publication: *Products of Excellence: ADA Seal Program* (list of ADA-accepted products)

Sjögren's Syndrome Foundation, Inc.
(see address/phone and fax numbers under Sjøgren's Syndrome)
Publication: *List of Products Frequently Used by People with Sjögren's Syndrome*

LUPUS ERYTHEMATOSUS

Lupus Foundation of America, Inc.
1300 Piccard Drive, Ste. 200, Rockville, MD 20850
1-301-670-9292; 1-800-558-0121
Offers: patient education and referrals to support groups throughout N. America

SJÖGREN'S SYNDROME

National Sjögren's Syndrome Association
21620 N. 19th Ave., A-8, Phoenix, AZ 85027
P.O. Box 4227 Phoenix, AZ 85080
1-602-433-9844; 1-800-395-6772
Offers: information on SS; also acts as a support group and liaison for patient-to-patient contact

Sjögren's Syndrome Foundation, Inc.
333 N. Broadway, Ste. 2000, Jericho, NY 11753
1-516-933-6365; 1-800-475-6473
fax: 1-516-933-6368
e-mail: ssf@mail.idt.net
Publications: newsletter *The Moisture Seekers®*; product list—see Clinical Products above

SYSTEMIC SCLEROSIS

Scleroderma Foundation
89 Newbury St., Ste. 201, Danvers, MA 01973
1-800-722-4673
fax: 1-978-750-9902
e-mail: sclerofed@aol.com
Internet: www.scleroderma.org
Offers: patient education packet and referrals to support groups throughout N. America; physician referral; research grants

Scleroderma International Foundation
704 Gardner Center Rd., New Castle, PA 16101
1-412-652-3109
Publication: newsletter, *The Connector*

Scleroderma Research Foundation
2320 Bath St., Ste. 315, Santa Barbara, CA 93105
1-800-441-CURE; 1-805-563-9133
Internet: www.srfcure.org
Offers: fund-raising for research grants and facilitation of research
Publications: *Scleroderma Research Foundation Newsletter*

Appendix B Diagnostic Tests

Tables 9 and 10 summarize many of the diagnostic tests pertaining to the six rheumatic diseases/syndromes discussed in this coursebook. These tests are only one step in the diagnostic process. Before making a diagnosis, clinicians should also consider: (1) patient history; (2) signs and symptoms; and (3) results of other tests. Many of the tests are done to exclude related disorders with similar clinical characteristics. Some of the tests are also used to monitor side effects of drugs prescribed to treat the disorders.

Table 9. Diagnostic Blood Tests

When testing for:	And finding:	Consider:
Antinuclear antibodies (ANAs),	• The presence of ANAs (the higher the titer, the greater the likelihood of disease) — specifically, high titers of:	RA, Sjögren's, SLE, or SSc
	• Anti-dsDNA	SLE
	• Anti-La/SS-B and/or anti-Ro/SS-A	Sjögren's or SLE
	• Anti-Sm	SLE
	• Antitopoismerose I	SSc
	• Anticentromere	SSc
	• Anti-RNA polymerases I, II, and/or III	SSc
Antiphospholipid antibodies	• Antibodies to cardiolipin or other phospholipids may result in a false-positive serologic test for syphilis, detection of a lupus anticoagulant, or artifactual prolongation of in vitro coagulation studies	SLE
CBC, including: • white blood count (WBC) • hemoglobin (HGB) • hematocrit (HCT) • platelet count	• Subnormal levels of any values at left, with a positive ANA test • Elevated WBC, which can indicate leukocytosis • Subnormal HGB or HCT, which can indicate anemia • Diminished platelet count, indicating thrombocytopenia	RA or SLE
Complement activity: total, CH_{50}; and C3 and C4 levels	• Subnormal levels of these proteins, indicating ongoing activation of the immune system	SLE
Creatinine	• Abnormally high levels of creatinine, which can indicate impairment of kidney function	RA, CFS, or SSc
Erythrocyte sedimentation rate (ESR) or C-reactive protein (CRP)	• An abnormally rapid rate, indicates an increase in blood protein, due to inflammation and/or infection. • The presence of CRP, which indicates inflammation.	RA
Liver enzymes	• Abnormally high levels of alanine aminotransferase may indicate diminished liver activity, hepatic inflammation, or medication toxicity (interpret test results cautiously).	RA or SLE
Nonagglutinating antibodies to red cells	• These antibodies (using the Coombs'/antiglobulin test) indicates autoimmune hemolytic anemia	SLE
Rheumatoid factor (RF)	• High titers of RF	RA or Sjögren's
Occult blood	• Blood (using the stool guaiac test), which suggests GI bleeding, perhaps indicative of medication toxicity	RA

Table 10. Basic Diagnostic Medical Tests		
To assess:	**In patients with:**	**Consider ordering:**
Bony structures	RA *(see Table 1)*	• Standard x-rays to detect changes and irregularities in joint alignment or contours
GI tract function	SSc *(see diagnostic tests, Chapter 5)*	• A barium swallow to detect esophageal hypomotility, gastroesophageal reflux, or gastrointestinal dysmotility
Iridocyclitis	JRA *(see pauciarticular JRA, Chapter 1)*	• A slit-lamp examination, which involves: 1. Emitting intense light through a lamp slit to illuminate the patient's eye 2. Inspecting the eye through a magnification scope *Normally, the light passes through the eye unimpeded, but, with inflammation, it is abnormally diffused.*
Lacrimal gland function	Sjögren's *(see Algorithm 9)*	• A Schirmer test for tears, which involves: 1. Inserting filter paper between the eyeball and the lower eyelid 2. Removing the filter paper *Normally, in 5 min, a young person moistens 15 mm of a paper strip; however, patients with SS may wet <5 mm in 5 min.*
Lung volume and pressure	SSc *(see diagnostic tests, Chapter 5)*	• A pulmonary function test, which involves: 1. Having the patient exhale, after a full inspiration, as hard and fast as possible into a spirometer 2. Recording the amount of air exhaled during the first second *This test shows the ability of the patient's lungs to exchange oxygen and carbon dioxide.*
Salivary gland function or inflammation	Sjögren's *(see Algorithm 9)*	• Salivary scintigraphy, which involves: 1. Administering I.V. radionuclide, which migrates to sites of inflammation, in one or more salivary glands 2. Observing and evaluating images obtained by a special camera • Parotid sialography, which involves radiographs of parotid salivary ducts
Synovia	RA *(see Table 1)*	• An arthrocentesis, which involves inserting a large aspirating needle into a joint to collect synovia *Diseased synovia is often cloudy yellow-green and contains numerous leukocytes; normal synovia is clear, pale yellow, and contains few cells.*
Tissue abnormalities and inflammation	SLE *(see renal biopsy, Chapter 3)* Sjögren's *(see Algorithm 9)* SSc *(see Algorithm 10)*	• Biopsy, which involves removing a small piece of living tissue for microscopic examination (e.g., biopsy of a minor salivary gland) • Radiograph or CAT scan of soft tissues of the lungs (e.g., to detect interstitial pulmonary fibrosis, or pulmonary alveolitis)
Urine abnormalities	*RA (see Table 1)* *CFS (see Table 4)* *SLE (see Algorithm 7)*	• Urinalysis, which involves examining urine, by microscope or dipstick, to detect abnormal amounts of serum proteins and/or abnormal numbers of blood cells in urine
Vascular changes	SSc *(see diagnostic tests, Chapter 5)*	• Nail-fold capillaroscopy, which involves examining nail-fold capillaries with a microscope or an ophthalmoscope

Post-Test

Note your answers on this post-test (to keep for your own reference) and on the answer form, using a #2 pencil. There is only one correct answer to each question. Please consult tables, graphs and their captions, and algorithms, as well as the text, for answers to the questions.

1. Most of the six rheumatic disorders can manifest ____.
   a. rapidly
   b. systemically
   c. occultly
   d. intermittently

2. A normal immune system works by producing ____.
   a. pathogens
   b. antigens
   c. antibodies
   d. leukocytes

3. ANAs are ____.
   a. desensitized lymphocytes
   b. foreign antigens
   c. spontaneous remissions
   d. circulating autoantibodies

4. Redness, heat, swelling, and pain are indications of ____
   a. inflammation
   b. hypomobility
   c. malaise
   d. autoimmunity

5. To diagnose systemic sclerosis, most physicians use criteria prepared by the ____.
   a. CFS
   b. ACR
   c. CDC
   d. AMA

6. RA is a(n) ____ disease which usually develops slowly.
   a. systemic
   b. chronic
   c. autoimmune
   d. all of the above

7. Of the 2.5 million adult RA patients in the United States, more are ____.
   a. men
   b. young
   c. women
   d. Chinese

8. When certain cells in the synovium's tissues proliferate, ____ is formed.
   a. a pannus
   b. subchondral bone
   c. a capsule
   d. joint cartilage

9. Typical radiographic evidence of RA usually shows ____.
   a. synovial effusion
   b. joint swelling
   c. subcutaneous nodules
   d. bone erosion

10. Structural damage caused by synovitis is ____.
    a. rare
    b. irreversible
    c. reversible
    d. extraarticular

11. Active synovitis does not usually cause pain in ____.
    a. the morning
    b. MCP joints
    c. wrist joints
    d. sacroiliac joints

12. Carpal tunnel syndrome causes pain, tingling, and ____ of the thumb.
    a. numbness
    b. deformity
    c. crepitus
    d. erosion

13. MTP joint arthritis can cause ____.
   a. burning paresthesia
   b. knee thickening
   c. cock-up toe deformity
   d. wrist deformity

14. TMJ pain may be a symptom of ____.
   a. muscular atrophy
   b. active synovitis
   c. ulnar deviation
   d. tarsal tunnel syndrome

15. Nodules developing in the fingers of RA patients are ____.
   a. Bouchard's nodes
   b. lumps of tissue
   c. spurs
   d. Heberden's nodes

16. JRA onset may be ____.
   a. pauciarticular
   b. polyarticular
   c. systemic
   d. all of the above

17. Spiking fever in late afternoon or evening indicates ____ JRA onset.
   a. systemic
   b. pauciarticular
   c. polyarticular
   d. RF-positive

18. Early treatment with ____ may change the course of RA.
   a. NSAIDs
   b. DMARDs
   c. glucocorticoids
   d. anticytokines

19. Neither CFS nor FMS is ____.
   a. controversial
   b. painful
   c. inflammatory
   d. disabling

20. Aside from chronic fatigue, patients must have at least 4 ____ to be diagnosed with CFS.
   a. sleep disorders
   b. tender nodes
   c. unusual headaches
   d. symptom criteria

21. A condition such as ____ excludes a diagnosis of unexplained CFS.
   a. bulimia
   b. rhinitis
   c. telangiectasia
   d. sarcoidosis

22. The drugs offering most benefit to CFS patients are ____.
   a. gamma globulins
   b. DMARDs
   c. NSAIDs
   d. tricyclic antidepressants

23. In FMS patients, high-frequency alpha waves interfere with ____.
   a. serum serotonin levels
   b. delta wave sleep
   c. tender point palpation
   d. alkaline phosphatase levels

24. Symptoms characterizing FMS include ____.
   a. fatigue
   b. stiffness
   c. pain
   d. all of the above

25. The age group in which incidence of SLE peaks is ____.
   a. 1 to 4 year olds
   b. 5 to 14 year olds
   c. 15 to 40 year olds
   d. 45 to 60 year olds

26. Over 95% of SLE patients have ____.
   a. chilblain lesions
   b. active glomerulonephritis
   c. serum ANAs
   d. discoid lesions

27. Antibodies to certain phospholipids in the blood serum of SLE patients may lead to a falsely positive serologic test for ____.
   a. nephritis
   b. syphilis
   c. pericarditis
   d. RA

28. In SLE patients with glomerulonephritis, the presence of chronic scarring and fibrosis may mean the disease is ____.
   a. inactive
   b. irreversible
   c. nonfatal
   d. infectious

29. Alopecia affecting patients with discoid lesions is ____.
   a. diffuse
   b. reversible
   c. permanent
   d. inflamed

30. ____ can trigger an SLE flare-up.
   a. sunlight
   b. stress
   c. pregnancy
   d. all of the above

31. NSAIDs are used to treat ____ in SLE patients.
   a. glomerulonephritis
   b. pleurisy
   c. strokes
   d. skin lesions

32. ____ is a major characteristic of Sjögren's syndrome.
   a. alopecia
   b. xerostomia
   c. candidiasis
   d. mucositis

33. A positive result on a parotid sialography test means the patient has ____.
   a. xerostomia symptoms
   b. KCS symptoms
   c. lacrimal gland shrinkage
   d. salivary gland involvement

34. The presence of Raynaud's phenomenon in a primary Sjögren's patient usually means ____ involvement.
   a. digit
   b. joint
   c. lung
   d. lymphoid

35. Sjögren's syndrome patients should avoid ____.
   a. salted pretzels
   b. milk products
   c. red meat
   d. raw vegetables

36. The microvascular injury caused by systemic sclerosis ____ the internal lining of small arteries.
   a. erodes
   b. thickens
   c. cracks
   d. indurates

37. The pathogenesis of systemic sclerosis may start with ____.
   a. an esophageal dysfunction
   b. congestive heart failure
   c. toxic oil syndrome
   d. an endothelial injury

38. A tendon friction rub indicates that ____ has affected the tendons.
   a. fibrosis
   b. fibromyalgia
   c. calcinosis
   d. anticentromere

39. The first phase of limited systemic sclerosis cutaneous involvement is ____.
   a. indurative
   b. atrophic
   c. edematous
   d. hypertrophic

40. Raynaud's phenomenon is an exaggerated response to ____.
   a. heat
   b. cold
   c. dampness
   d. sunlight

41. Sclerodactyly is caused by the replacement of fatty tissues with ____.
   a. calcium
   b. fluid
   c. capillaries
   d. collagen

42. The main cause of death for systemic sclerosis patients is ____.
   a. arterial blockage
   b. pulmonary disease
   c. renal crisis
   d. intestinal dysmotility

43. D-penicillamine is fairly effective therapy for ____.
   a. cutaneous fibrosis
   b. pulmonary fibrosis
   c. renal crisis
   d. pulmonary hypertension

44. Methotrexate, a(an) ____ is often the initial DMARD given to patients with severe RA.
   a. calcium channel blocker
   b. antimalarial agent
   c. antimetabolite
   d. ACE inhibitor

45. ____ is a safer alternative to other DMARDs.
   a. Sulfasalazine
   b. Methotrexate
   c. D-penicillamine
   d. Azathioprine

46. Patients on long-term glucocorticoid therapy should ____.
   a. be closely monitored
   b. wear medical alert bracelets
   c. have dosing regimens altered
   d. all of the above

47. Surgery patients with cardiac defects may need prophylactic antibiotics to prevent ____.
   a. pulmonary hypertension
   b. bacterial endocarditis
   c. gastrointestinal bleeding
   d. renal insufficiency

48. Cold applied to pain receptors acts as a(n) ____.
   a. stimulant
   b. analgesic
   c. irritant
   d. tranquilizer

49. Eating ____ benefits patients with rheumatic diseases.
   a. sweet potatoes
   b. oily fish
   c. cooked fruits
   d. baked chicken

50. To keep joints from becoming stiff and deformed, ____ exercises are recommended.
   a. strengthening
   b. aerobic
   c. high impact
   d. range of motion

Transfer your answers to the answer form by filling in the appropriate letter <u>using a #2 pencil</u>. Verify that your name and the course title are on the answer form. <u>Request your certificate by completing the form on the next page.</u>

Index

Reference List for Further Study

1. Weyand CM, Goronzy JJ. Pathogenesis of rheumatoid arthritis. In: Snyderman R, Haynes BF, guest eds. *Advances in Rheumatology.* The Medical Clinics of North America. Philadelphia, PA: WB Saunders Co. January 1997;81(1):29-55.
2. Kwoh CK, Simms RW, et al. Guidelines for the management of rheumatoid arthritis. *Arthritis Rheum.* May 1996;39(5):713-722.
3. Rothschild BM, Woods RJ. Symmetrical erosive disease in Archaic Indians: the origin of rheumatoid arthritis in the New World? *Sem Arthritis Rheum.* 1990; 19:278-284.
4. Benedek TG. History of the rheumatic diseases. Chap 1 in: Schumacher HR, ed. *Primer on the Rheumatic Diseases.* 10th ed. Atlanta, GA: Arthritis Foundation. 1993.
5. Winchester R. Rheumatoid arthritis. Vol II, chap 38 in: Frank MM, Austen KF, Claman HN, Unanue ER. *Samter's Immunologic Diseases.* 5th ed. Boston, MA: Little, Brown & Co. 1995.
6. Arthritis Foundation. *Rheumatoid Arthritis.* Publication 835-5320. Atlanta, GA. June 1996.
7. Wilder RL. Rheumatoid arthritis: epidemiology, pathology, and pathogenesis. Chap 10, sec A in: Schumacher HR, ed. *Primer on the Rheumatic Diseases.* 10th ed. Atlanta, GA: Arthritis Foundation. 1993.
8. Rosenberg AE. Skeletal system and soft tissue tumors. Chap 27 in: Cotran RS, Kumar V, Robbins SL. *Robbins Pathologic Basis of Disease.* 5th ed. Philadelphia, PA: WB Saunders Co. 1994.
9. Arnett FC, Edworthy SM, Bloch DA, et al. The American Rheumatism Association 1987 revised criteria for the classification of rheumatoid arthritis. *Arthritis Rheum.* March 1988;31(3):315-324.
10. Anderson RJ. Rheumatoid arthritis: clinical features and laboratory. Chap 10, sec B in: Schumacher HR, ed. *Primer on the Rheumatic Diseases.* 10th ed. Atlanta, GA: Arthritis Foundation. 1993.
11. Shmerling RH, Fuchs HA, et al. Guidelines for the initial evaluation of the adult patient with acute musculoskeletal symptoms. *Arthritis Rheum.* January 1996;39(1):1-8.
12. Arthritis Foundation. *Carpal Tunnel Syndrome.* Publication 835-5225. Atlanta, GA. March 1996.
13. Ball G, Koopman W. Rheumatoid arthritis. Chap 154 in: Kelley WN, editor-in-chief. *Textbook of Internal Medicine.* Philadelphia, PA: JB Lippincott Co. 1989.
14. Williams HJ. Rheumatoid arthritis: treatment. Chap 10, sec C in: Schumacher HR, ed. *Primer on the Rheumatic Diseases.* 10th ed. Atlanta, GA: Arthritis Foundation. 1993.
15. Cassidy JT, et al. A study of classification criteria for a diagnosis of juvenile rheumatoid arthritis. *Arthritis Rheum.* 1986;29:274.
16. Singsen BH. Pediatric rheumatic diseases: nonarticular rheumatism, juvenile rheumatoid arthritis, juvenile spondylarthropathies. Chap 22, sec A in: Schumacher HR, ed. *Primer on the Rheumatic Diseases.* 10th ed. Atlanta, GA: Arthritis Foundation. 1993.
17. Arthritis Foundation. *Arthritis in Children.* Publication 835-5415. Atlanta, GA. April 1996.
18. Grom AA, Glass DN. Juvenile rheumatoid arthritis. Vol II, chap 39 in: Frank MM, Austen KF, Claman HN, Unanue ER. *Samter's Immunologic Diseases.* 5th ed. Boston, MA: Little, Brown & Co. 1995.
19. Malawista S, Hardin J. Rheumatoid arthritis. Vol 1, sec 5-14 in: *Clinical Dermatology.* Philadelphia, PA: Harper and Row. 1985.
20. Pearson MH, Rönning O, Odont D. Lesions of the mandibular condyle in juvenile chronic arthritis. *Br J Orthodontics.* 1996;23:49-56.
21. Van der Heijde DM, van Riel PL, Nuver-Zwart IH, et al. Effects of hydroxychloroquine and sulfasalazine on progression of joint damage in rheumatoid arthritis. *Lancet.* 1989;1:1036-1038.

22. Van der Heide A, Jacobs JWG, Bijlsma JWJ, et al. The effectiveness of early treatment with "second-line" antirheumatic drugs: a randomized, controlled trial. *Ann Intern Med.* 1996:124:699-707.
23. Kirwan JR and the Arthritis and Rheumatism Council Low-Dose Glucocorticoid Study Group. The effect of glucocorticoids on joint destruction in rheumatoid arthritis. *N Engl J Med.* 1995;333:142-146.
24. Jain R, Lipsky PE. Treatment of rheumatoid arthritis. In: Snyderman R, Haynes BF, guest eds. *Advances in Rheumatology.* The Medical Clinics of North America. Philadelphia, PA: WB Saunders Co. January 1997;81(1):57-84.
25. Moreland LW, Baumgartner SW, Schiff MH, et al. Treatment of rheumatoid arthritis with a recombinant human tumor necrosis factor receptor (p75)—Fc fusion protein. *N Engl J Med.* July 17, 1997;337(3):141-147.
26. Firestein GS, Zvaifler NJ. Anticytokine therapy in rheumatoid arthritis. *N Engl J Med.* July 17, 1997;337(3):195-197.
27. Brandt KD, Slemenda CW. Osteoarthritis: epidemiology, pathology, and pathogenesis. Chap 24, sec A in: Schumacher HR, ed. *Primer on the Rheumatic Diseases.* 10th ed. Atlanta, GA: Arthritis Foundation. 1993.
28. Moskowitz RW, Goldberg VM. Osteoarthritis: clinical features and treatment. Chap 24, sec B in: Schumacher HR, ed. *Primer on the Rheumatic Diseases.* 10th ed. Atlanta, GA: Arthritis Foundation. 1993.
29. Mahowald ML. Infectious arthritis: bacterial agents. Chap 26, sec A in: Schumacher HR, ed. *Primer on the Rheumatic Diseases.* 10th ed. Atlanta, GA: Arthritis Foundation. 1993.
30. Naides SJ. Infectious arthritis: viral and less common agents. Chap 26, sec B in: Schumacher HR, ed. *Primer on the Rheumatic Diseases.* 10th ed. Atlanta, GA: Arthritis Foundation. 1993.
31. Krey PR. Arthropathies associated with hematologic diseases and malignant disorders. Chap 35 in: Schumacher HR, ed. *Primer on the Rheumatic Diseases.* 10th ed. Atlanta, GA: Arthritis Foundation. 1993.
32. Guzman L. Rheumatic fever. Chap 21 in: Schumacher HR, ed. *Primer on the Rheumatic Diseases.* 10th ed. Atlanta, GA: Arthritis Foundation. 1993.
33. Fan PT, Yu DTY. Seronegative spondylarthropathies: Reiter's syndrome. Chap 20, sec C, in: Schumacher HR, ed. *Primer on the Rheumatic Diseases.* 10th ed. Atlanta, GA: Arthritis Foundation. 1993.
34. Taurog JD. Seronegative spondylarthropathies: epidemiology, pathology, and pathogenesis. Chap 20, sec A, in: Schumacher HR, ed. *Primer on the Rheumatic Diseases.* 10th ed. Atlanta, GA: Arthritis Foundation. 1993.
35. Khan MA. Seronegative spondylarthropathies: ankylosing spondylitis. Chap 20, sec B, in: Schumacher HR, ed. *Primer on the Rheumatic Diseases.* 10th ed. Atlanta, GA: Arthritis Foundation. 1993.
36. Kroenke K. Chronic fatigue: frequency, causes, evaluation, and management. *Comprehensive Ther.* 1989;15:3-7.
37. Fukuda K, Straus SE, Hickie I, et al. The chronic fatigue syndrome: a comprehensive approach to its definition and study. *Ann Intern Med.* December 15, 1994;121(12):953-939.
38. Shafron SD. The chronic fatigue syndrome. *Am J Med.* 1991;90:730-739.
39. Klonoff DF. Chronic fatigue syndrome. *Clin Infectious Dis.* 1992;15:812-823.
40. Arthritis Foundation. *Fibromyalgia.* Atlanta, GA. February 1992.
41. Yunus MB. Fibromyalgia syndrome: new research on an old malady. *Br Med J.* 1989;298:474-475.
42. Smythe HA, Moldofsky H. Two contributions to understanding of the "fibrositis" syndrome. *Bull Rheum Dis.* 1977;28:925-931.
43. Wolfe F, Smythe HA, Yunus MB et al. The American College of Rheumatology 1990 criteria for the classification of fibromyalgia: report of the multicenter criteria committee. *Arthritis Rheum.* February 1990;33(2):160-172.
44. Freundlich B, Leventhal L. The fibromyalgia syndrome. Chap 41 in: Schumacher HR, ed. *Primer on the Rheumatic Diseases.* 10th ed. Atlanta, GA: Arthritis Foundation. 1993.
45. Clauw DJ. Fibromyalgia: more than just a musculoskeletal disease. *Am Family Physician.* September 1, 1995; 52(3):843-851.

46. Wilke WS. Fibromyalgia: recognizing and addressing the multiple interrelated factors. *Postgraduate Med.* July 1996;100(1):153-170.
47. Buchwald D, Garrity D. Comparison of patients with chronic fatigue syndrome, fibromyalgia, and multiple chemical sensitivities. *Arch Intern Med.* 1994;154:2049-2053.
48. Goldenberg D, Mayskiy M, Mossey C, et al. A randomized, double-blind crossover trial of fluoxetine and amitriptyline in the treatment of fibromyalgia. *Arthritis Rheum.* November 1996;39(11):1852-1859.
49. Russell IJ, Fletcher EM, Michalek JE, et al. Treatment of primary fibrosis/fibromyalgia syndrome with ibuprofen and alprazolam: a double-blind, placebo-controlled study. *Arthritis Rheum.* 1991;35:552-560.
50. Cotran RS, Kumar V, Robbins SL. Diseases of immunity. Chap 6 in: Cotran RS, Kumar V, Robbins SL. *Robbins Pathologic Basis of Disease.* 5th ed. Philadelphia, PA: WB Saunders Co. 1994.
51. Kotzin BL, O'Dell JR. Systemic lupus erythematosus. Vol II, chap 37 in: Frank MM, Austen KF, Claman HN, Unanue ER. *Samter's Immunologic Diseases.* 5th ed. Boston, MA: Little, Brown & Co. 1995.
52. Arthritis Foundation. *Lupus.* Publication 835-5245. Atlanta, GA. April 1996.
53. Benedek TG. Historical background of discoid and SLE. Chap 1, sec 1 in: Wallace DJ, Hahn BH, eds. *Dubois' Lupus Erythematosus.* 5th ed. Baltimore, MD: Williams & Wilkins. 1997.
54. Pisetsky DS. Systemic lupus erythematosus: epidemiology, pathology, and pathogenesis. Chap 11, sec A, in: Schumacher HR, ed. *Primer on the Rheumatic Diseases.* 10th ed. Atlanta, GA: Arthritis Foundation. 1993.
55. White P. Pediatric rheumatic diseases: other pediatric rheumatic diseases. Chap 22, sec C, in Schumacher HR, ed. *Primer on the Rheumatic Diseases.* 10th ed. Atlanta, GA: Arthritis Foundation. 1993.
56. Schur PH. Clinical features of SLE. Vol 2, chap 61 in: Kelley WN, Harris ED Jr, Ruddy S, Sledge CB. *Textbook of Rheumatology.* 4th ed. Philadelphia, PA: WB Saunders Co. 1993.
57. Belmont HM, Abramson SB, Lie JT. Pathology and pathogenesis of vascular injury in systemic lupus erythematosus. *Arthritis Rheum.* January 1996;39(1):9-22.
58. Quismorio FP, Jr. Other serologic abnormalities in SLE. Chap 31 in: Wallace DJ, Hahn BH, eds. *Dubois' Lupus Erythematosus.* 5th ed. Baltimore, MD: Williams & Wilkins. 1997.
59. Pisetsky DS, Gilkeson G, St. Clair EW. Systemic lupus erythematosus: diagnosis and treatment. In: Snyderman R, Haynes BF, guest eds. *Advances in Rheumatology.* The Medical Clinics of North America. Philadelphia, PA: WB Saunders Co. January 1997;81(1):113-128.
60. Gladman DD, Urowitz MB. Systemic lupus erythematosus: clinical features. Chap 11, sec B in: Schumacher HR, ed. *Primer on the Rheumatic Diseases.* 10th ed. Atlanta, GA: Arthritis Foundation. 1993.
61. Wallace DJ. Cutaneous and cutaneovascular manifestations of SLE. Chap 39, sec VI in: Wallace DJ, Hahn BH, eds. *Dubois' Lupus Erythematosus.* 5th ed. Baltimore, MD: Williams & Wilkins. 1997.
62. Rhodus NL, Johnson DK. The prevalence of oral manifestations of systemic lupus erythematosus. *Quintessence Int.* 1990;21(6):461-465.
63. Marino C. Oral lesions and connective tissue diseases. *DMD: A Dentist's Medical Digest.* December 1989;XI(12):2-3.
64. Brown RS, Flaitz CM, Hays GL, et al. The diagnosis and treatment of discoid lupus erythematosus with oral manifestations only: a case report. *Compend Contin Educ Dent.* June 1994;XV(6):724732.
65. Ward MM, Pyun E, Studenski S. Mortality associated with specific clinical manifestations of systemic lupus erythematosus. *Arch Intern Med.* June 24, 1996;156(12):1337-1344.
66. Petri M. Pathogenesis and treatment of the antiphospholipid antibody syndrome. In: Snyderman R, Haynes BF, guest eds. *Advances in Rheumatology.* The Medical Clinics of North America. Philadelphia, PA: WB Saunders Co. January 1997;81(1):151-177.
67. Klippel JH. Systemic lupus erythematosus: treatment. Chap 11, sec C in: Schumacher HR, ed. *Primer on the Rheumatic Diseases.* 10th ed. Atlanta, GA: Arthritis Foundation. 1993.
68. Moutsopoulos HM. Sjögren's syndrome. Chap 15 in: Schumacher HR, ed. *Primer on the Rheumatic Diseases.* 10th ed. Atlanta, GA: Arthritis Foundation. 1993.

69. Kruize AA, Hené RJ, van der Heide A, et al. Long-term follow-up of patients with Sjögren's syndrome. *Arthritis Rheum.* February 1996;39(2):297-303.
70. Talal N. Sjögren's syndrome and connective tissue diseases associated with other immunologic disorders. Vol 2, chap 78 in: McCarty DJ, Koopman WJ, eds. *Arthritis and Allied Conditions: A Textbook of Rheumatology.* 12th ed. Philadelphia, PA: Lea and Febiger. 1993.
71. Arthritis Foundation. *Sjögren's Syndrome.* Publication 835-5330. Atlanta, GA. April 1996.
72. Carsons S. Distinguishing primary from secondary. In: *Sjögren's Syndrome.* Port Washington, NY: Sjögren's Syndrome Foundation. 1994.
73. Gobetti JP, Froeschle ML. Sjögren's syndrome: a challenge for dentistry. *General Dentistry.* May-June 1997.
74. Udell I. Dry eye (keratoconjunctivitis sicca). In: *Sjögren's Syndrome.* Port Washington, NY: Sjögren's Syndrome Foundation. 1994.
75. Atkinson JC, Wu AJ. Salivary gland dysfunction: causes, symptoms, treatment. *JADA.* April 1994;125:409-416.
76. Atkinson JC, Fox PC. Sjögren's syndrome: oral and dental considerations. *JADA.* March 1993;124:74-86.
77. Mitchell H, Bolster MB, LeRoy EC. Scleroderma and related conditions. In: Snyderman R, Haynes BF, guest eds. *Advances in Rheumatology.* The Medical Clinics of North America. Philadelphia, PA: WB Saunders Co. January 1997;81(1):129-149.
78. Silver RM. Systemic sclerosis (scleroderma). Vol II, chap 42 in: Frank MM, Austen KF, Claman HN, Unanue ER. *Samter's Immunologic Diseases.* 5th ed. Boston, MA: Little, Brown & Co. 1995.
79. Denton CP, Black CM, Korn JH, De Crombrugghe B. Systemic sclerosis: current pathogenetic concepts and future prospects for targeted therapy. *Lancet.* May 25, 1996;347(9013):1453-1458.
80. Silman AJ, Black CM, Welsh KI. Epidemiology, demographics, and genetics. In: Clements PJ, Furst DE, eds. *Systemic Sclerosis.* Baltimore, MD: Williams & Wilkins. 1996.
81. Silver RM. Scleroderma and pseudoscleroderma: environmental exposures. In: Clements PJ, Furst DE, eds. *Systemic Sclerosis.* Baltimore, MD: Williams & Wilkins. 1996.
82. Steen VD, Medsger TA Jr. The palpable tendon friction rub: an important physical examination finding in patients with systemic sclerosis. *Arthritis Rheum.* June 1997;40(6):1146-1151.
83. Medsger TA Jr, Steen V. Systemic sclerosis and related syndromes: clinical features and treatment. Chap 13, sec B in: Schumacher HR, ed. *Primer on the Rheumatic Diseases.* 10th ed. Atlanta, GA: Arthritis Foundation. 1993.
84. Pisetsky DS, with Trien SF. *The Duke University Medical Center Book of Arthritis.* New York, NY: Fawcett Columbine Books. 1992.
85. Herrick AL, Oogarah PK, Freemont AJ, et al. Vasculitis in patients with systemic sclerosis and severe digital ischaemia requiring amputation. *Annals Rheumatic Dis.* May 1994;53(5):323-326.
86. Nagy G, Kovacs J, Zeher M, et al. Analysis of the oral manifestations of systemic sclerosis. *Oral Surg Oral Med Oral Pathol.* February 1994;77:141-146.
87. Parma-Benfenati S, Ferreira PA, Fugazzotto PA, et al. Progressive systemic sclerosis (scleroderma): oral-mucosal changes. *General Dentistry.* March-April 1986:107-112.
88. Nylor WP. Oral management of the scleroderma patient. *JADA.* 1982;105(5):814-817.
89. Steen VD. Organ involvement: renal. In: Clements PJ, Furst DE, eds. *Systemic Sclerosis.* Baltimore, MD: Williams & Wilkins. 1996.
90. Rosenthal AK, McLaughlin JK, Gridley G, Nyren O. Incidence of cancer among patients with systemic sclerosis. *Cancer.* Sept. 1, 1995;76(5):910-914.
91. Steen VD, Lanz JK, Conte C, et al. Therapy for severe interstitial lung disease in systemic sclerosis: a retrospective study. *Arthritis Rheum.* 1994;37:1290-1296.
92. Rich S, Kaufman E, Levy PS. The effect of high doses of calcium channel blockers on survival in primary pulmonary hypertension. *N Engl J Med.* 1992;327:76-81.
93. Simms RW, Kwoh CK. Guidelines for monitoring drug therapy in rheumatoid arthritis. *Arthritis Rheum.* May 1996;39(5):723-731.
94. Wilkins EM. Care of patients with disabilities. Chap 50 in: Wilkins EM. *Clinical Practice of the Dental Hygienist.* 7th ed. Malvern, PA: Williams & Wilkins. 1994.